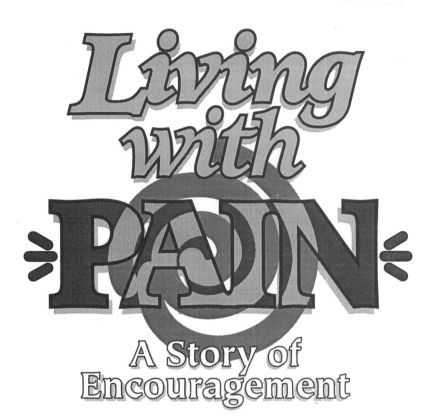

Living with PAIN

A Story of Encouragement

Dr. Samuel C. Gipp

Friend to Churches Publishers

ISBN 1-890120-02-2
Library of Congress Catalog Card No. 96-090983

⁖ by
Bible and Literature Missionary Foundation
713 Cannon Blvd.
Shelbyville, TN 37160

By the Same Author

- A Practical and Theological Study
  of the Book of Acts
- An Understandable History of the Bible
- The Answer Book
- Job
- Answers to the Ravings of a Mad Plunger
- Is the Holy Spirit Female?
- Reading and Understanding the Variations
  Between the Critical Apparatuses of
  Nestle's 25th and 26th Editions of
  the Novum Testamentum-Graece

Future Releases

- A Practical and Theological Study
  of the Book of John
- How to Minister to Youth
- Selected Sermons (Volumes 1–10)

Order from
Friend to Churches Publishers
P. O. Box 587
Northfield, Ohio 44067-0587
(800) 311-1823

Foreword

Just about everybody suffers from some sort of pain, and everybody's pain is different. As excruciating as mine is, it can be defined by the most important word there is when dealing with permanent pain . . . **bearable**.

But that is not due to what might be perceived as an insignificant amount of pain. I believe that enduring constant pain entails both the mental and spiritual condition of the person in question.

As a rule I tend to be a "Non-depressant" type of person. I've always been pretty light hearted and jovial. This has helped immensely in dealing with my pain.

I also have an unshakable faith in the Lord Jesus Christ and the infallibility of the Bible. This is what has taken me beyond that which is capable with only medication and a good attitude. If you have not yet received Jesus Christ as your personal Saviour you not only have abandon your greatest ally in your battle with pain, but you have left your soul in the precarious position of going to a Christless eternity, where **no book** on pain relief will be able to help you.

Reading this book does not guarantee you victory in your battle with pain. But having Jesus Christ as your personal Saviour does.

"And he said unto me, My grace is sufficient for thee: for my strength is made perfect in weakness. Most gladly therefore will I rather glory in my infirmities, that the power of Christ may rest upon me" (2 Corinthians 12:9).

Contents

1

How It Happened

I laid there on a pile of broken concrete blocks, bent nails and small pieces of two-by-fours looking two floors up at the stairwell opening through which I had just fallen. Blood oozed from a gaping wound in the back of my head, several ribs were fractured and though I did not know it at the time . . . **my neck was broken**. It was the beginning of a long journey that would lead to a life in which pain was to be a constant companion and adversary. A life where my faith in Jesus Christ and His Bible would be all that got me through.

> **Blood oozed from a gaping wound in the back of my head, several ribs were fractured and though I didn't know it at the time . . . my neck was broken!**

It was August 23, 1973. A little over three years earlier, on June 14, 1970, I had gone forward in the College and Career Class of the Canton Baptist Temple, in Canton, Ohio, and trusted Jesus Christ as my personal Saviour. This is quite an experience for anyone, but for a twenty year, Roman Catholic, drunkard it was absolutely life changing! Ten short weeks later found me in Pensacola, Florida attending the Pensacola Bible Institute preparing for the ministry. A mere three months had passed since I had graduated from Bible college and entered the field of evangelism. Furthermore, it was less than two weeks since the August 12th date of the first anniversary of my marriage to the former Kathaleen Fay Vaughan.

Now I lay in an unfinished basement, in a pool of my own blood. It was a day that I would be reminded of everyday for the rest of my life because of the pain that would accompany me throughout the days of rest of my life.

Just a Normal Day

This day had started out as normally as any other. As a young evangelist of twenty-three years old and just out of Bible college, I had taken a job working for a construction company owned by a Christian man. He allowed me to take time off so that I could take meetings when I had them, but still provided a job when I had no meetings. I had spent that morning driving a dump truck. We were hauling rock to be used in the foundation of a new house. Strangely, sitting in the cab of the truck while it was being weighed, I noticed a safety sign posted on the weight shack that showed a man falling and read, "Watch out for

What I thought was standing up, was in fact a two story back swan dive down through the stairwell opening into the basement.

falls!" I thought it interesting that this sign had caught my attention, since others had consistently gone unnoticed.

Later that day I was at a different building site. Here we had already raised the walls of the first floor of a another new house and decked the second floor. Now we were building the walls for the second story in preparation of raising them also. We had laid the two-by-fours on edge for the frame work of the front wall and nailed them together. Next we nailed the sheathing to the outer side of the walls. At the ends we would nail on four-by-eight sheets of plywood which would add strength to the structure. After this we would raise the wall, nail it to the

> ## If he had simply adjusted my neck he would have killed me!

second floor and then fabricate the remaining outside walls. I was at the end of the wall, on top of a piece of half-inch plywood that would act as a brace for the corner. I was on my hands and knees nailing the plywood on as I slowly backed up, working from the outer edge of the house toward the center. As I felt my feet come over the edge of the top of the wall I was on, I went to stand up. I thought that I was only about 4 inches off the floor. I was wrong! I hadn't thought to turn around and look behind me or I would have seen that I had been backing toward the opening where the stairs would later go. It was on open hole, two stories down. At the bottom was the pile of broken concrete blocks, bent nails and odd pieces of wood which were swept down there at the end of each working day.

As my feet came over the top edge of the wall I stood up, or so I thought. What I thought was standing up, was in fact a two story back swan dive down through the stairwell opening and into the basement. I can still remember falling. I remember seeing a coworker on the first floor looking up from lighting a cigarette as I fell passed him. As I fell I remember thinking, "Gipp, This is the **STUUUUUUPIDEST** thing you've ever done." I hit the edge of the first floor as I fell past it. The impact from this split my skull and most likely broke neck. Then I crashed down onto the pile of rumble that lay in the basement, breaking several ribs.

I laid there, amazed that I was still conscious. I looked two floors up to see my fellow workers peering down at me over the edge of the opening. A ladder was lowered and I stood up to climb out. A mistake! As soon as I stood up I passed out from shock and was laid back down by my worker friends to await an ambulance.

I was rushed to the nearest hospital and admitted, X-rayed and shot full of the appropriate medications. A foam cervical collar was put around my neck to help support my head. Later that afternoon, when the pain of the fall was just catching up to me an Indian doctor entered my room. He was the emergency room doctor who had admitted me. He asked how I felt and I told him I was OK except for the pain I felt and the numbness in my arms. I asked what the X-rays had showed. He told me that I had broken a few ribs (As though I didn't know!) and said that the X-rays

> **As I bent over to remove my t-shirt, the doctor quickly stopped me with a worried look on his face and said with a touch of terror in his voice, "Don't bend over!"**

revealed that something was wrong with my neck. "But," he said, "I've turned you over to your regular doctor and he will be taking care that." (That's what he thought!)

My wife Kathy, who is a Licensed Practical Nurse, watched this doctor as he filled out the admittance form. She saw him write, "Check for possible cervical fracture" (broken neck).

It may seem amazing, but in spite of the X-rays and the Emergency Room doctor's comments, **my personal doctor overlooked my broken neck**. Just four days after the fall I was released from the hospital. Due to my broken ribs I didn't go back to work until two weeks later . . . **with my neck still broken!**

A Shocking Revelation

The next two months were filled with misery. I experienced pain in my neck and arms accompanied by reoccurring numbness. I returned to my doctor to tell him of this, only to be treated like a hypochondriac. During what was to be my last visit to this man I insisted that he do something about the pain and numbness that I was experiencing in my arms. His exact words were, "I'll give you some **green pills**. Try the bathtub and hot water." Then he walked out to his nurse and said something to her. She opened a drawer in her desk and handed me a box of "green pills." Two months of fruitless appeals had led to this. I walked out of his office in anger and told my wife, "Now we're going to a **real** doctor." With that, we headed for a chiropractor.

> **Sam, you should be paralyzed from the neck down!**

We went to a man of good reputation who was also a member of our church. None of us knew it at the time, but if he had simply adjusted my neck he would have killed me. But this doctor refused to treat a neck injury without first taking X-rays. After X-raying my neck he led me into his examination room and asked, "Has anyone ever told you that you have a broken neck?"

I, ever appreciative of a good one liner, said, "Not this week!"

Rather than laugh at my joke he said, "Well you've got one!"

He then placed one of my X-rays on the examination screen. Before he could point to my injury, I saw that one of the vertebrae in my neck was bent down at about a 45 degree angle while all the rest of them stood straight out.

He pointed out the damage and explained that I had a break between my C6 and C7 vertebrae. I asked him what he would be doing to treat this problem. He

> **My neck was repaired, but something was wrong—I couldn't talk!**

stated, "I've already called an orthopedic surgeon. You are going straight there from here. You are now his patient . . . and Sam, **walk carefully**."

Kathy and I arrived at the specialist's office, a Dr. Smith, with our heads spinning from the sudden turn of events. The surgeon looked at the chiropractor's X-rays and also the original ones that the hospital took on the day I fell. They were identical. Yet, for his own safety, he wanted to take his own. He asked me to remove my shirt so I could be X-rayed. As I bent over to remove my T-shirt, the doctor quickly stopped me with a worried look on his face and said with a touch of terror in voice, "**Don't bend over!**" With this one single statement it slowly began to dawn on me that I was into something bigger than I ever had been before.

With a puzzled expression I asked, "Why?"

Dr. Smith said solemnly, "Sam, you should be paralyzed from the neck down from the fall you took. But from walking around for two months, you should be **dead**! If you had nailed over your head in the last two months it would have killed you."

With these words I remembered the **many times** that I had nailed over my head in the preceding two months. I remembered driving one of the company dump trucks to the land fill and **bouncing off the head liner** with my head. I realized then that the hand of my gracious God had been protecting me from a terrible fate.

The doctor examined me and made urgent arrangements to get me admitted to the hospital. (A **different** hospital than the one I went to after the fall.) He reported that there would be no room available for two more weeks. Kathy and I went cautiously home. Upon our arrival the telephone rang. It was Dr. Smith. He had pulled every string possible and gotten me admitted in the hospital scheduled for the next day.

The following day, November 5th I was admitted and immediately I was put in cervical traction. To do this two holes were drilled into the sides of my head and what looked like a small set of stainless steel ice tongs was screwed into the holes. A rope with twenty pounds of weight was then attached to the tongs. I laid in bed in traction like this for seven days. Then on November 12th I was taken into surgery. 81 days had passed since my accident.

The procedure performed on me is now common. It is called "Cervical Fusion." The front of my throat was cut and a hole was drilled into the vertebrae that encompassed the broken vertebrae and a good one. Then a 5/8" plug of bone was removed from my right hip and inserted into this opening. Eventually the bones would grow together and secure the broken vertebrae. My broken neck was now repaired. But things were not "fine."

> **I finally came to the realization that pain was to be a permanent part of my life.**

Several hours later I awoke in the Recovery Room to find my wife waiting anxiously beside me. The operation had been a success. My neck was repaired. But something was wrong? **I couldn't talk!**

The doctors soon realized that during the surgery my vocal cords had contracted. I could speak in only a hoarse whisper. The "evangelist" had his body back, but had lost the ability to **preach**! It would be four long months before God graciously restored my voice. It still gives me problems today, but it has served me, and Him, well for several decades. I have no complaints.

The problem with the pain that I experience today is due primarily to the length of time that passed between the breaking of my neck and getting it repaired. You can imagine, for example, if you broke your leg and then didn't get it set for almost three months. Your leg would never heal as well as if it had been set immediately. That is what is wrong today with my neck.

How Not to Get Rich

You are probably wondering about a law suit. Yes, there was one. I am not a vindictive person by nature. Nor am I interested in a "windfall" profit. My wife and I had several people urge us to sue the doctor who had overlooked my broken neck and then ignored my pleas for help. We prayed about this and told the Lord that He would have to tell us if He wanted us to sue this doctor. If we did, we planned on dividing the money into fourths. Three of whose segments were to be sent to three individual missionaries and the fourth we would keep for ourselves. We told the Lord that He would have to make it **plain** to us that He wanted us to sue.

Two days later, the lawyer that we had contacted to help file my Workman's Compensation forms called. He said that the surgeon who had operated on my neck had called him and advised us to sue our doctor. With that we initiated a suit. Please bear in mind that this was 1973, not 1993. If it had been 1993, there would have been any number of slick lawyers with television ads that would promise to sue the breeches of a mother for serving her child cold cereal. And they would win. In 1973 it was not so. My workman's compensation lawyer made the arrangements. I ended up meeting a lawyer from Cleveland, Ohio at the **train station** in Canton, Ohio. We talked briefly while he looked at his watch. He took my box of "green pills." I never saw him, or them, again. A few weeks later I was informed that "I" had decided to settle out of court. I few weeks after that I received my check. What would doubtless have netted *five million* dollars in 1993 ended up being *five thousand* dollars in 1973. We paid the lawyer, tithed, then split the money into fourths. We sent our three missionaries their money and kept the remaining fourth. It came to about one thousand dollars.

I've included the information about the law suit because today such blatant **legitimate** malpractice would net the victim millions of dollars. Therefore, people reading this book might think that was what happened in my case. It didn't. Due to my injury I was unable to work for a year. During that year the state of Ohio's department of workman's compensation paid us $52 a week to live on. After tithing, that was less than $50. Our share of the settlement was soon gone. We have no regrets. God took care of us.

Slow Light Dawning

I spent the year after my release from the hospital wearing a brace that extended from my waste to my chin in front and the base of my skull in the back. During this period I also underwent physical therapy, A year after my surgery I was released to go back to work. I resumed my endeavors in the field of evangelism where I had left them a year previous. I thought that I would put the entire issue of my broken neck behind me and start over. But I soon found that was not to be.

As I stated earlier. Due to the period of time that passed between my actual injury and the corrective surgery, my neck has never completely returned to normal. Somewhere there are still "a few crossed wires"!

This truth was very slow in dawning on me. I had expected to experience a little bit of pain following my surgery. The discomfort I experienced during my year of recuperation didn't alarm me either. In fact, as I dutifully submitted to every kind of remedy that was offered or suggested I fully expected that something would stop the pain. It was not until over **ten years** had passed that I finally came to the realization that pain was to be a permanent part of my life. There would be days when it would be rather benign. There would be days when it would be vicious. There would be days when it would threatened my sanity. But, no matter what its manifestation, it would be my constant companion for the rest of my life.

2

One Visitor, Many Guises

I have lived with pain for nearly a quarter of a century now. Although my pain is constant, it differs almost daily in how it will afflict me. Understandably, some days are better than others, yet everyday is visited by unremitting pain in some form.

To better convey the experience of daily pain I have cataloged the many varieties of pain that make a regular appearance in my life.

> **Just when you feel that you have learned to live with this daily, accepted discomfort, you learn a disheartening thing— somedays the rock seems bigger!**

There's a Stone In My Shoe

I am now more than twenty years removed from that hot August day in 1973, yet it is always, unwillingly close to me. I am reminded of it everyday, for I never go through a day without some sort of pain due to that accident. The pain is always there. Some days it is a minor irritation. Sometimes it is a great burden. In spite of this I have found that you can adjust to pain. You don't necessarily get used to it. But you can adjust to it. There is a certain amount of pain that I have everyday. I view the daily "normal" everyday pain that I feel in my neck as though it were a small stone in my shoe.

Imagine that you had a small stone in your shoe that you couldn't remove. Believe it or not, after a while you would adjust to it. You would no longer be surprised or angered by its presence. You would learn how to step so as not to aggravate the problem. You would resign yourself to those things that you just couldn't do anymore, like say; running. But you would eventually learn to live with it. You would soon accept this small irritation as "normal."

> **You have to "retrain" your brain to ignore a higher level of discomfort.**

That is how I go through each day. I wake up every morning with pain in my neck. I go to sleep each night the same way. But I have even found that sleep is not an escape, as I am frequently awakened during the night by a sharp stab of pain in my neck. Yet over the years I have come to accept this daily discomfort as "normal." To this day when someone asks me if my neck hurts and all I have is "the stone in my shoe" I reply that I am not hurting. I'm not lying. I simply mean, "I have no more than my normal daily pain."

Unfortunately, just when you feel that you have learned to live with this daily, accepted discomfort, you learn a disheartening thing. Some days **the rock seems bigger**! On those days when the rock seems small you can actually get used to ignoring it. You simply learn to operate with a constant amount of discomfort. Your mind is condition to ignore this "normal" pain. Then one day you find that the rock has gotten bigger and consequently, harder to ignore. Now you are forced to start all over again with this new problem. You have to "retrain" your brain to ignore a higher level of discomfort. You learn that there are new restrictions to what you are able to do.

> **I go through the day feeling like a pit bulldog has snapped his jaws closed on the back of my neck and just hangs there all day.**

Over the years I have learned to deal with these restrictions. For example, I have found that when I sit in a room and talk to people that I can't keep my head turned to the right very long without the pain becoming overbearing. So when I sit in a room I try to find a seat that will be exactly opposite the person that I will be speaking to. This is a simple adjustment but it makes a great difference in my personal comfort. I don't regularly ask concessions to my pain from those around me. But I make some small ones myself that are covert such as this.

I have also found that I have a problem sitting in church. This problem arises from the height and angle from where I'm sitting to the pulpit. If I sit too far off to the side I am forced to turn my head sideways and my neck ends up hurting. The same thing is true if I sit so close that I must constantly look up. For these reasons I am careful to get a seat that is close to the center of the auditorium and about half way back. This way I can look just about straight ahead at the preacher. This may seem like an insignificant thing but it helps me to keep the size of the "stone in my shoe" small.

There can be a sadness to avoiding pain. One of the sadder things for me is that I have to be careful of hugging children. Sometimes a well meaning child will give me a "bear" hug which quickly becomes an "**unbearable**" hug for me. It's an awful feeling to have a child locked on to your neck as you feel sheets of pain course through your neck and you have to try to smile and not scream. I have also had an occasional overzealous brother give me a hug that put me out of commission for a several days. The sad part of this is that you can't walk around saying, "Don't hug me!" to anyone that comes near. Instead of this, you try to avoid the unwanted situation at the expense of looking unsociable.

> There are times that I will be reading and then look up just to have a bolt of pain shoot down my neck.

The Pit Bull

There are some days that I experience what I call "The Pit Bull." This is where I go through the day feeling like a pit bulldog has snapped his jaws closed on the back of my neck and just hangs there all day while I go about my business. You can imagine the "slight" discomfort that this would be!

The "Pit Bull" is a dull pain which is usually accompanied by some slight shooting pains when I turn or lift my head. The "stone" is an **everyday** situation and I don't take any pain killers for it. The "Pit Bull" usually lasts a whole day and can be with me for several. I don't take anything for this pain either until it has been with me for too many days and I am tired of it. I'm not brave. The fact is simply that I have enough of what I consider "serious pain" that **requires** medication. If I took a pain killer **every time** I had pain that was more serious than "The Stone," I would be a junkie.

The "Pit Bull" will always be accompanied by sharp shooting pains that are caused by turning or raising my head too quickly. You wouldn't believe how many times I've absent mindedly shaken my head only to feel "the Bull" clamp on tighter and just about send me through the ceiling. There are times that I will be reading and then look up just to have a bolt of pain shoot down my neck.

As I said, I usually don't treat "The Pit Bull" with pain killers. Rather than using pain killers, I treat "the Pit Bull" with heat. (More on that later.) If I apply heat to my neck early in the day I am sometimes able to make "the Bull" release its grip, leaving me to contend with no more than a "stone" in my shoe.

The Ax and the Knife

There are other days that I get out of bed feeling like someone has just walked up behind me and buried an ax between my shoulder blades. I turn to see the cause of my discomfort only to see him turn and say, "Have a nice day!" as he walks away.

"The Ax" will usually be accompanied by numbness in a couple of fingers or aching pains in one or both of my forearms. There have been times when I have even had the sensation that a fly was walking on the back of my hand. Yet when I look I see nothing though I can still feel it.

> **Sometimes I can almost feel the blade of "the Ax" as though it was a physical object sticking in my back.**

"The Ax" tends to immobilize me to a small degree. It is impossible to sit or stand in a position that relieves the pain. I find some relief from the discomfort if I hold my head up and back. This produces a slight "nose high" attitude. But it also provides some relief. When I am being afflicted by "The Ax" I am unable to bow my head for prayer. This may look arrogant or unhumble to a viewer, but it is a necessity to me.

18

Sometimes I can almost feel the blade of "The Ax" as though it was a physical object sticking in my back, right between my shoulder blades, just to the left of my spine. (As it is doing while I write this!) Sometimes it even makes my ribs ache so that I can honestly say, "It only hurts when I breathe."

> ## With "the Knife" comes the initial stages of immobility.

The most common treatment which I use on "The Ax" is "The Buffer." "The Buffer" is a big two handed vibrator that I have. Because the pain is located in the middle of my back, I have to lay on my stomach on a bed and let Kathy "buff" my shoulders and neck. I usually try not to take any pain killers for "The Ax." You learn to live with a certain amount of pain, even if that certain amount grows bigger on some days.

"The Knife" is similar to "The Ax" but with characteristics that merit an individual title. "The Knife" obviously feels like I have a knife in my back rather than an ax. But what makes "The Knife" different is its location. This is the sensation of having a knife turned sideways and driven directly between vertebras C6 and C7 in the back of my neck. "The Knife" will get your attention! I don't know if the guy who drives "the Knife" into my neck as the same one who buries "The Ax" in my back. But, **for sure**, his aim is just as good!

Along with "The Knife" come some **very sharp pains** (no pun intended) when I move my head. Of all of the manifestations that my pain employs, "The Knife" is one of the least common but extremely severe. With "The Knife" comes the initial stages of immobility. I tend to turn from the waste to look side-to-side rather than from the neck. Sometimes I simply cannot turn to talk to someone. I will just tell the person that I'm sitting in a room speaking with to disregard the fact that I am talking to them but looking straight ahead.

Thankfully "The Knife" doesn't seem to stay around for much more than a day or two. I usually treat it with heat and "The Buffer." If it is coincident with "The Ax" I'll take a couple of aspirins also.

Froze Up!

Sometimes due to making the wrong move or sleeping in a bad position I will feel a little "Pop!" in my neck. Beside the intense shot of pain that accompanies this, it is the harbinger of what is coming. I know that I am going to be experiencing what I call being "Froze Up" or "Locked Up." The circumstances of this situation is an inability to turn my head very far without searing pain shooting through it. My neck is too stiff to move without great discomfort.

Probably one of the most remarkable things about some of the "sieges" of pain that I have is that it takes no great effort on my part to cause them. I have long ago stopped lifting anything heavy if I have any choice in the matter. Yet, next to sleeping and cold weather, which I will deal with later, most problems begin with just the slightest turn of the head. I remember vividly one Sunday morning, just before going into a church to preach that I turned my head to the left to say something to my wife. Suddenly there was the now familiar "Pop!" in my neck along with a lightning bolt of pain.

> **By the time I was finished with the morning services I could no longer move my head.**

Then I was fine, but I looked at my wife and said, "I've got about an hour before I 'lock up'." I went into the church and taught Sunday School. Even while I spoke I could "feel the cement hardening" in my neck. By the time I was finished with the morning services I could no longer move my head.

When this condition arises I know that I am in for a "siege" of intense pain and discomfort that will last for a minimum of three days and a maximum of about three weeks. Sometimes when I'm "froze up" I can't turn my head . . . period! My wife will often have to support my head to help me lay down or sit up in bed. I will roll over in my sleep only to awake with a cry as a bolt of pain explodes in my neck.

> **I can feel a fly walking on the back of my hands, yet when I look, there is nothing.**

As though the pain was not enough, this condition leads to some very embarrassing situations when I'm preaching. Since I am an evangelist, I am usually preaching **somewhere** almost every night. I have never yet canceled a service due to pain or immobility. More times than I can count I have been preaching while "froze up." Suddenly the slightest move will trigger a lightning bolt of pain and I will cry out involuntarily. I feel like an absolute "Jerk" when this happens, but I am determined to fulfill my call to preach, pain or no pain.

There are times when I am "froze up" that I can't turn my head well enough to drive. I will let Kathy drive while I plant my head firmly against the head rest of the passenger seat to keep from being jostled around by the movement of our van. We live in a 35 foot long travel trailer that we pull with a 1 ton Ford conversion van. Many times turning a corner will set up a rocking motion that will almost destroy me if I'm already "froze up." There have been many times that this sudden rocking motion of the van has triggered a siege of being "froze up" when I hadn't been experiencing any serious problems. (It's called "Life in the Fast lane.") Sometimes the rocking of the van as we cross an uneven set of railroad tracks will do the same thing.

Periodically, being "froze up," will be accompanied by little "explosions" of pain up and down the length of my arms. Being "Froze Up" is occasionally accompanied by that sensation of having a fly walking around on the back of my hand or arm. It is amazing how I can feel that fly walking on the back of my hands, yet when I look, there is nothing. Yet, even while I'm looking I can feel them walking!

I usually pull out all of the stops when trying to end the pain of one of these sieges. I take aspirins, apply heat, and use "The Buffer." There have been times when I've spent hours laying in bed with a heating pad under my neck. Occasionally I have spent most of the day lying on a heating pad, then I go in the church and preach, and then return immediately to the trailer and lay back down on the heating pad. But eventually my neck loosens up and I resume normal operations.

> **If your pain gets the better of your mind, you're in big trouble.**

Broken Glass and Gravel

Have you ever heard the sound of gravel crunching under the tire of a car on concrete? That is the sound I hear whenever I turn my head. Some days seem worse than others. There is no pain associated with this. But the sound is grating. There have been times when I've half expected to hear that sound and then go limp for the rest of my life.

Head Pain

Some of the most unbearable times come when my head hurts as a result of my neck being "out." Everything that I've talked about so far starts at my neck and goes down. **Down** my back. **Down** my shoulders. **Down** my arms. But head pain occurs when the pain decides to go **up** as well. It usually starts at the base of my skull and proceeds to slowly expand until it encompasses my entire head. There will be spots of pain that are more intense than others. Sometimes it's the back of my head. Sometimes the front. At other times one of the sides of my head will ache with tremendous pain.

When my neck is "out" I can experience head pain for as long as two weeks. When added to the assorted pains previously mentioned, the situation can become pretty "intense." The headaches are absolutely agonizing. It hurts to read. It hurts to work. It almost hurts to **think**!

> **My constant desire is to open the door and run out into the night. To find a place where I can hide. But I can't "hide" from my neck!**

I write books, work up new sermons and formulate Bible studies to be taught as lessons in Sunday School classes in the churches where I preach. When I experience the other pains I can pretty well continue to work. When the pain of a neck generated headache is added in I am almost useless. I simply cannot concentrate on the subject at hand at the same time that I am trying to endure a barrage of pain. Sometimes taking a few aspirins and sleeping for about an hour will at least improve the situation to where I can work again. At other times, pain killers won't even touch it.

It may be hard to believe, but as intense as these contests with pain become, I have been able to endure them fairly well. I am resolved to the experience of pain as a normal (for me) part of my life. Yet there are times when it undeniably borders on unbearable. There are two conditions where the onslaught of pain is almost victorious. In both of these instances the attack is on the mind. All pain is in fact, an attack on the mind. **If your pain gets the better of your mind, you're in big trouble.**

Cabin Fever

The condition that I call "Cabin Fever" is not unlike the "Cabin Fever" that people suffer from during a particularly hard winter. It is a psychological condition and manifests itself as panic. As winter progresses, some people begin to feel closed in by it and feel a need to escape. They feel that they are prisoners of their houses and realize that there will be no rescue from this feeling until the spring thaw. This leads directly to a panicked feeling of not being able to "escape" winter. This condition can become very serious, yet can be relieved by nothing more than an unseasonably warm weekend in December or a desperate flight to Florida for a few days. Though I am mentally unaffected by the severity or length of winter, I do experience a "Cabin Fever" of my own.

My "Cabin Fever" also arises from a mental need to escape. Unfortunately, what I need to escape from is **pain**. An escape that will not come in this world.

> **The bottom line on pain is: You must deal with it (and win!) alone.**

Most often "Cabin Fever" will occur in the middle of the night. Many times after I've been awakened by neck pain due to sleeping in the wrong position or from turning my head in my sleep. More than once I've moved wrong in my sleep and woke up crying out in pain in the middle of the night. Many times I can't get comfortable enough to get back to sleep. As I lay there in the dark I come face to face with the grime reality that I will never have a day, or night, without pain. I feel an almost overwhelming desire to open the trailer door and **run!** But I realize that anywhere I go **I will take my neck with me** and therefore, my pain. The desperation is almost suffocating! My constant desire is to open the door and run out into the night. To find a place where I can hide. **But I can't "hide" from my neck!** I will have no sooner fought off one of these almost irresistible urges to escape the inescapable when another wave will wash over me. It takes a very great deal of prayer and all of the mental control that I can exert to remain immobile. My wife is a wonderful woman and tremendously patient with my problems. During an attack of "Cabin Fever" I am afraid I will awaken her. I don't want to over load her capacity for sympathy. The bottom line on pain is: You must deal with it (and win!) alone.

> You cannot imagine the feeling of having endured days of pain and then finally to feel that it is over, only to have it lay off for one day and then return again the next with a vengeance.

Although most attacks of "Cabin Fever" come at night, there are times when there is even no safety to be found in the brightness of the day. Sometimes when I have been enduring an unusually long siege of extreme pain, that one word will unexpectedly flash through my mind; "Escape!" Fortunately I am a realist concerning my pain and have learned to accept what I can do nothing to change. But the bouts with "Cabin Fever" will take me to the edge to my mental endurance. They are not pleasant. They are not romantic. They are both **real** and **frightening!**

Torture

The other attack that weakens the resolve to continue on is a

---

[1] I remember on one occasion of dreaming of taking pain killers only to wake up that morning with a monstrous headache that stayed with me for three days.

condition that I call "Torture."

The act of torture is an attack on the **mind** not the body even though the body is the recipient of the punishment. You are tortured by an enemy in order to break down your resolve. To destroy your resistance. The principle is simple; "I'm going to hurt you until you do what I want you to do." When faced with the anticipation of torture, the mind automatically "braces up" for whatever is to come. Once the assault on the body is over and the prisoner is returned to his cell, the mind tends to relax. The cruelest technique of torture comes at this time. Just as the prisoner feels that he has endured the abuse of his tormentor and has emerged victorious he is **immediately taken back in for another "session."** Just when the mind thought that it had endured and prevailed, and so had begun to relax, it is subjected to the punishment again. This feeling of never being allowed to relax from the torment will **break** the human will.

My "Torture" is very similar to this. It starts with a grueling siege of pain that will last from ten days to two weeks. The pain will manifest itself in every form conceivable. During this time I will be subjected to any or all of the above described phases of pain. I will have days when I can't move my head. I will spend days with "The Pit Bull" hanging onto my neck while "The Ax" is sticking in my back. I will be forced to endure little starbursts of pain up and down my arms. I will pop aspirins, "buff" my back and head until the skin is sore, and spend *days* on the heating pad. Many times my neck is so fragile that even my Bible is too heavy for me to carry without aggravating the problem and must be carried to my preaching services by one of my sons. During this time I will wake up with a start from moving wrong in my sleep. I will wake up with extreme pain and go to sleep the same way. I have even experienced the pain in my dreams![1]

Finally, after days and nights of unrelenting pain, I will

notice one day that the pain is passing. I'm almost hesitate to acknowledge it because of the fear of being wrong. But, sure enough, something in my neck has gotten right and the pain will begin to dissipate. I will feel like a wrung out dish rag, but joyful that I have endured. My arms won't hurt. My head won't hurt. My neck will ache a bit which is really "normal." It is like having the sun come out after a terrible storm. Like silence after a tremendously loud buzzing noise. I will be able to move my head again. My mind will relax . . . and then the next day, **the pain is back!**

You cannot imagine the feeling of having endured *days* of pain and then finally to feel that it is over, only to have it lay off for one day and then return again the next with a vengeance. It is the only time that tears come to my eyes. It is when I just don't think that I can take anymore.

Sometimes I equate trying to live with constant pain and not going crazy to walking a tightrope. Walking a tightrope is something that is hard enough to do as it is. When "the Torture" hits I feel like someone is shaking the rope.

The most important thing that you can do during "the Torture" is to resolve yourself **not to give in.** If you are "broken" by your pain, then you are a defeated individual. A slave.

Hiroshima—the Day After

There is one great truth about the pain. **It will pass sometime!** It may not go away completely, but it will either recede to a point where it is bearable, or you will adjust to it to a point of being able to endure it better.

Trying to live a normal life without allowing the pain to run it taxes both the mind and body. When I have endured an extended assault by pain I am thankful when it is passed. But I am quite often both emotionally and physically **drained.** Have you ever seen that famous picture of Hiroshima, Japan on August 7, 1945? That is the day **after** they dropped the

27

atomic bomb. It is a picture of utter devastation. That picture is how I feel after enduring a long siege of pain. Basically, I need about a day to get it all back together. After periods that are not so severe or so long I feel like a worn out punching bag or a wrung out dish rag. But if it has been **intense** and **prolonged**, it is Hiroshima.

I'm Miserable. It's Wonderful!

I experience pain in some form, to some degree everyday of my life. The names that I have ascribed to the various manifestations of pain best describe the way they affect me. As you can see, some are undoubtedly worse than others. For this reason I find days that I can describe as **merely** miserable much better than the days that I find to be almost **unbearable**. I have found myself thankful for the lesser pain and more than willing to endure it as long as the "heavy stuff" stays away.

3

Cause and Effect

If you have a stone in your shoe that cannot be removed, the easiest way to stop the pain is to simply **not walk**. A "pain in the neck" is not the same. Unfortunately, the pain that I experience in my neck is going to be there no matter what I do. There are some precautions though that I can take in an attempt not to aggravate the problem.

As can be expected, I don't make a habit of lifting heavy items. Although you don't lift with your neck, you do strain it when you lift. This is especially true if you are carrying something that is heavy and then turn your head to look around for a place to put it down. This means that I have long ago given up on helping to move anyone's refrigerator! There are times while setting up our trailer at a church where I will be preaching that I am forced to carry the trailer hitch from the van to a shed or basement room. During these times I am extremely careful in every movement that I make. But the fact is, I have long ago swallowed my pride. I usually ask anyone who happens to be there at the time if they have back problems. If they don't, I request that they carry the hitch for me. It is **a lot** easier that hurting!

Ya Gotta Sleep Sometime!

Sadly, there are a few things that you simply can not influence or alter in life. One of these is; **sleep.**

Sleep is inescapable. Everybody has to sleep. Yet sleeping is one of the worst things I can do for my neck. The reason is obvious. I will assume a position while sleeping that will cause me to wake up with a stiff neck. For me, a stiff neck in the morning is not something that passes by noon. It usually develops into being "Froze up" or a three day long headache. Many times my wife has awaken in the middle of the night to find me sleeping with my head cocked to one side or laying off of the pillow. She will gingerly lift my head back onto my pillow and hope that I haven't already caused myself tomorrow's grief. Sometimes I have awakened to find that my neck is stiff and sore from the position in which I was sleeping. I will mumble something to myself like, "Tomorrow should be a 'fun' day." and then nod back off to sleep and wait to see what the morning will bring. Most of the time, it brings nothing good.

> You can imagine how the next day is when it is a combination of pain and sleepless exhaustion.

There are other times when a sudden movement in my sleep has caused me to sit straight up in bed yelling out in pain. Then the trouble is immediate! I have spent some torturous nights in which I nod off only to be awaken by pain about every twenty or thirty minutes. You can imagine how the next day is when it is a combination of pain and sleepless exhaustion. But don't worry. You live through them.

Cold—A Bitter Enemy

I was born in northeastern Ohio and was therefore raised in

winters full of ice and snow. I have always enjoyed winter. Such things as, shoveling snow, plowing snow and ice skating were not unusual. Even today, I am not a "winter hater." But the years have added a new factor, a broken neck. I have been diagnosed as having arthritis in my neck. This has made winter time anything **but** something to look forward to with joyful anticipation. Winter for me is one long siege. I am an unwilling prisoner of our little travel trailer throughout the winter, until the warmth of summer comes. My wife and I try to walk about three miles everyday. Yet in the winter, I dare not walk or else I am faced with the prospect of spending several hours with a heating pad wrapped around my neck in an attempt to get some pain out, and some movement back into it.

> We have awakened to have so much ice on the inside of our trailer door that we couldn't open it.

Living all year long in a little travel trailer has lent itself to some unique situations in the battle with pain. One of the singly most effective things that I can do to get heat back into my neck is to fill a bathtub with hot water and soak my neck for about an hour. True, finding yourself sweating for an hour after your bath is not pleasant, but at least this achieves the desired effect on my neck. My simple problem is this, you can't sit down in the size of bathtub that a is found in a trailer bathroom. The bathtub in our trailer is 38 inches long and only 17 inches wide. These are not the proportions necessary to submerge a full grown adult. Even if the tub was large enough to sit in, our six gallon hot water heater would hardly produce enough hot water to **warm** a whole tub of water let alone **heat** one. Therefore, my most effective deterrent to cold weather is unattainable.

Trailer life also makes for unique sleeping arrangements during the winter. A trailer is no more than a **glorified tent**. Heating one is little different from heating a tent. It heats up slowly and cools down **very quickly**. When the winter weather gets serious, it is almost impossible to get or stay warm in a trailer. This is especially true at night. We have endured temperatures down to 10 degrees below zero in our trailer. It was anything but pleasant. When winter arrives, I make it a regular practice to sleep with a turtle neck dickie on to help keep some heat in my neck. When the temperature really drops I go to bed looking very much like I'm about to embark on a trip to the North Pole. I wear socks, sweat pants,

> **Aging is an opponent that is harder to stop than George Foreman.**

a long sleeve turtle neck shirt, a sweater and a wool toboggan hat. We have awakened to have so much ice on the **inside** of our trailer door that we couldn't open it. I've had to direct a small electric heater at the door to melt the ice so that we could open it! There has been ice on our bedroom ceiling. Also we've had clothes frozen to closet walls. Once our bed was so cold that **it hurt** to lay on it. The next day we went out and bought an electric blanket to put **under** the sheet. It is needless to say that I spend a lot of time during the winter too stiff to move my neck well. But I'm blessed if I'm only miserable!

During the winter I will seldom attempt trips outdoors. If I do go out I bundle my neck up as much as possible to keep the heat in and the cold out. Sometimes there is repair work to do on the trailer during the winter. When this happens I may be forced to be outside for a long period of time. When I am outside like this I can feel the cold as it creeps into my neck. I will immediately apply some heat to my neck when I get back inside.

Don't Look!

One of the simplest and most foolish things that I do to hurt my neck is to simply turn my head to look at something. This is especially dangerous if I turn quickly. Even the simple act of responding to an inquiry in the negative with a quick shake of the head can lead to trouble. The problem is that such movements don't **always** cause a problem. Therefore, after hurting myself this way, I will be careful for a short while. Then I will get more relaxed and soon forget to be cautious. All this with no adverse effect. Then one day, the slightest quick movement to the right or the left will leave me temporarily crippled again.

There are times when I will be sitting in a chair and I will tilt my head straight back to kiss my wife who is standing next to me. Then I realize that lifting the weight of my head back up is going to cause me grief. My wife kisses me, then places her hand under my head and gently returns it to it full "upright and locked position."

Just Don't Get Old

One thing that none of us can do anything about is the fact that we are **all** getting older. The Bible says, "And as it is appointed unto men once to die, but after this the judgment" (Hebrews 9:27). With each passing day we come closer to agreeing with God in everything. The process of aging is unavoidable. Therefore whatever physical problem you face today will inevitably be a greater problem ten years from now if the Lord tarries His coming that much longer.

> **When you find something that helps you fight pain and aids your mobility, you have taken a giant step in a positive direction!**

I know of no one who has any kind of physical affliction that has gained more relief with age. The opposite is always true. Chronic problems simply become more chronic with age. Those confined to wheel chairs or beds fight greater battles with bedsores and muscle deterioration. Nerves, I think, are like wires. Overload them on a regular basis and they begin to get brittle and frayed. They don't take the abuse as well as they once did. Add to that the "blessing" of arthritis in the case of bone ailments and you find that aging is an opponent that is harder to stop than George Foreman.

Your goal should be to find those things that you can do that will help you to deal with your pain yet they don't make you a servant to a dying body for the rest of your life! Aging is relentless, but you must not give up.

Heat Is a Wonderful Thing!

Even during the summer, a cool night can have me unable to move my head very well. Since soaking in a hot tub is out of the question, the next best thing is "portable heat." As I have already mentioned, I spend a good deal of time during the winter with an electric heating pad laying on the back of my neck in an effort to get some heat put back into the bones. Some time ago my wife bought me a neck warmer that can be heated in a microwave oven. It looks like a tube sock that has been filled with a granular substance and then sewn closed and then had a little loop rope handle attached to each end. Three minutes in the microwave and it gives an hour's worth of heat. The advantage of this over the electric heating pad is that I can put on my coat and then wrap the neck warmer around my neck and go outside. If we have to drive on a cold day I can wear the neck warmer around my neck for the first hour which gives the van time to warm-up. You may consider this a minor thing, but when you find something that helps you fight pain and aids your mobility, you have taken a giant step in a positive direction!

There are some occasions when we end up staying in a

hotel for one or more nights rather than our trailer. I always try to take advantage of having a full size tub to soak my neck. An hour in a tub can stop **days** of pain dead in its tracks. In spite of this, I don't ask for or accept offers to use the bathtub of someone in a church where we might be preaching. It is simply too awkward to do no matter how helpful someone may wish to be. I have to deal with pain everyday, therefore one thing that I refuse to do is to make my pain the subject of attention or conversation. I simply am not

> **"Father, if You want me to have pain all of the time I accept it."**

going to go around begging bathtubs from people and then let my wife and children keep them occupied while I soak. Then face them all as I leave the bathroom only to have someone ask, "How do you feel?" "I feel miserable, you Idiot! Now talk about something else."

Many people, with good intentions, almost force their help on you if they know that you have a physical problem. I do not talk publicly about my pain. It is **not** open to discussion. There are times that I am with my close friends in which the subject may come up. But I resent and reject attempts by folks to casually discuss it. And offers of help, though well intentioned, are not accepted.

I Love Football—TWICE!

I was born and raised in Massillon, Ohio, the birthplace of professional football. Our **high school** football stadium seats 26,000 people. The late Paul Brown, founder of the Cleveland Browns and the Cincinnati Bengals professional football teams was at one time the coach of the Washington High School "Massillon Tigers." Earl Bruce, a successful former football coach at Ohio State University also coached at Washington High. Chris Spielman, the fierce lineman of the Detroit Lions is a former "Massillon Tiger." When you come from Massillon, Ohio, you learn football early and love it all of your life.

Although I was too small to play high school football in high school, I did play a lot of "sand lot" football with the other guys from my neighborhood. Sometimes, when we couldn't find anyone with a football, we all trekked out to the old baseball diamond and simply tackled each other. Though I now make it a point not to be so caught up with football that I ignore the serious things of life, I still enjoy watching a game now and then. We have no television in our trailer or van, so I usually only see an occasional game of football at our relatives' houses during the holidays.

One of the things that I've always loved about football is the opportunity to hit or be hit . . . **hard!**. It has always been a wonderful feeling to spring off the line and crack into the opponent facing you. I still have trouble with a knee that I tore up as the result of a sand lot football injury.

Yet there is a second reason that I love football. Back in 1973 when I had my cervical fusion, I asked my doctor if I would be able to continue to play football after the surgery. He said that there was no reason that I shouldn't be able to continue to enjoy my participation in the game that I loved so much. (Since then, a

> **I heard a crack in my neck like the sound of a two-by-four snapping in half.**

professional boxer who suffered a broken neck in a car wreck has returned to the ring following his fusion.) For years after that, with the assurance of my doctor, I enjoyed **many** a football game. During my years as a youth director I enjoyed "racking and cracking" the young men in my class in sand-lot games of football. **Tackle** football. **Real** football.

Nine years after my surgery I took the pastorate of a church in rural, upstate New York. Long before I went there they had instituted a men's prayer meeting every Saturday at 7:00 P.M. After my arrival we added a 6:00 P.M. football game just before the prayer meeting. **Tackle** football. **Real** football.

I had begun to experience problems with chronic pain in my neck and arms within about five years after my surgery. My right arm was the most severely affected by pain and a tendency to go limp. I was still certain at this time that the pain would someday pass and everything would be all right. By 1984 the pain had become unbearable. I would experience severe pain as many as twenty to twenty-five days out of each month. I could be sitting quietly when suddenly a lightning bolt of pain would shoot up my right arm, from the elbow to the right hand. There was no warning. No way of preparing for it. It would just **strike**. There was a gnawing pain in my neck and right arm. Some days I would sit for hours in my office doing little more than rubbing my arms in agony. I had tried everything imaginable to stop the pain. Chiropractic adjustment, therapy, portable traction, but nothing had worked. finally one day in my office at church I prayed this prayer; "Father, if You want me to have pain all of the time I accept it. But **this pain** is going to drive me insane. Then I'll be no good to You, me or anyone else."

Shortly after that prayer I was involved in one of our regular Saturday night football games. Although I loved playing on the line, I was just as happy to run the ball. Hitting and getting hit never sparked the slightest fear in me. On the proverbial "last play of the game" I was called on to do an end run. I broke free and headed straight for the goal line and the winning touchdown. Right on the goal line I was hit by an opposing player. As I went down, I spun around backwards so that my inertia would allow me to fall into the end zone for the touchdown. As I was falling backwards, off balanced and defenseless one of the men of the church hit me full force from the opposite side. I heard a crack in my neck like the sound of a two-by-four snapping in half. A thousand needles stabbed into my left arm. My left arm was numb and semi-paralyzed. I laid on my back writhing in pain for two or three minutes until the pain subsided enough for me to regain my composure. Then I informed the sad faced men looking down at me that I thought that I may have broken my neck again.

I was gingerly placed in a car and taken to the local hospital. Four hours later, X-rays revealed that my neck was **not** broken. The resident doctor determined that I had stoved my neck badly and that I would feel the effects of it for quite a few weeks. The accident happened on June 30, 1984. It wasn't until September of that year that the middle and index fingers on my left hand finally regained any feeling in them.

It was some time after this that I slowly came to the realization that the injury had altered something in my neck. I noticed that I no longer had the shooting pains in my right arm. The numbness was also gone. In fact, from that day to this, (twelve years) I have experienced that severe degree of pain in my arms only about a dozen times! The Lord had "adjusted" my neck! Sadly, since I am not going to fool around with a good thing, that football game was my last football game. It's not that I'm afraid of getting hurt. I just don't want to "mess with success." I could cry when I think of how much I miss playing football. Although I enjoy watching collegiate or professional football, I can't stand to watch a sand lot game. I want to be involved. But **I do so thank God** for answering my prayer and saving my sanity! He had allowed that football game to do for me what all the doctors and treatments had failed to do.

I **still** thank God from time to time for allowing that football game to relieve me of the unbearable pain I had been experiencing.

4

Remedies and Treatments

I do not make a habit of talking to people in public conversation about my pain. Talking to someone candidly about a physical problem is embarrassing to that individual. I have found that it is hard enough to have to deal with **real**, physical pain everyday. Having to make it a part of my conversational life also, would only surrender that much more time to it. That would be more than I could bear. Yet it is inevitable that people find out. Once they do, you are in for a life time of amateur doctors who have the cure for everything right there in their back pocket. **All of them mean well.** Over the years I have tried what the doctors advised, what friends suggested and what just seemed to make good sense. Following are some of the helpful and not so helpful hints that I have received over the years.

The Doctors

I was placed in traction a week prior to my cervical fusion. It is possible that was not long enough to make sure that no nerves were still pinched in my neck. I don't know. One of the first treatments that my doctor offered to alleviate the chronic pain in my neck and arms was traction. I was given a home traction unit. It consisted of a harness that fit under the chin, a rope that went over a small pulley that attached to the top of a door and a plastic bag that was to be filled with enough water to reach the desired weight. I must say that, if there was anything that never worked, it was the traction. No amount of water or time seemed to make even a

> **If you become preoccupied with the pain, you will slowly find that you have become a servant to it.**

slight change in my condition. I still have the traction unit. Someplace! I hope my life never depends on my finding it quickly. Especially since it is stored in an attic in Ohio and I am out of the state preaching most of the time.

I am **not** saying that, if *you* have a neck problem, traction may not help. Different things may work for different types of problems. I always recommend at least trying it.

I have also tried therapy on my neck. In the early years, immediately following my surgery, I went to my doctor's hospital for neck exercises. These also failed to eliminate the pain. I tried various things that my doctor suggested, but all to no avail.

Next I again tried going to a chiropractor. By this time I was pastoring the church in upstate New York so I was unable to return to the chiropractor that had originally found my broken neck. The chiropractor in New York was not of the "rack 'em and crack 'em" school. He had a hand held device that looked like a little stainless steel syringe. It was spring loaded. He placed it on "the trouble spot" and impacted it with a little plunger that shot from the end of the syringe. In my case he may as well have been hitting concrete. It had no effect whatsoever. After about a year he gave up on this approach.

The next thing that this man wanted to try was to rig me up with a little battery pack that hung on my waist that had wires that ran to points on my neck. These wires carried electrical current. The theory was that electrical impulses from the battery pack for neutralize the pain. There were two problems with this electronic wonder.

The first problem was that it was an unreliable and cumbersome system. We never could get the right "frequency" that would counteract the pain in my neck. Add to that the fact that I was expected to walk around with **wires taped to my neck**! Subtle! Very subtle! I felt like a side show freak wearing this thing.

The second problem was that I found the philosophy behind this treatment unacceptable. I wanted to treat **the problem**, my broken neck. This treatment was aimed at treating **the effect**, the pain. You cannot focus on the pain. If you become preoccupied with **the pain**, you will slowly find that you have become a **servant** to it. I had no intention of having this happen. We gave up on this attempt also, which hadn't been working anyway. I eventually quit seeing this doctor.

About this time I had my "football adjustment" which did what no doctor or treatment had been able to do. It corrected what was an apparent misalignment in my neck. I **still**

> **I don't want to end up a quadriplegic because of a simple neck adjustment.**

benefit from this occasion and praise the Lord constantly for His grace in making the adjustment but not allowing any serious injury. As I have already mentioned, I quit playing football after this because I didn't want to do anything that would send me back to "the bad old days." More fearfully, I realized that I had moved something in my neck that was not supposed to be movable. I figure that if "the immovable" can be moved once, it can move twice, possibly with less than positive results the next time. For this reason I won't allow a chiropractor to adjust my neck. I don't want to end up a quadriplegic because of a simple neck adjustment. Maybe it would happen. Maybe it wouldn't. I am not taking any chances!

Once, many years later while I was holding a meeting in the Seattle, Washington area, I heard about a doctor who had a unique treatment for neck problems. I went to him since I had been experiencing problems in my neck that were above the cervical fusion point and I thought he might be able to help.

The treatment session took only about a half an hour, although the time at the office stretched out to eight hours due to orientation classes, X-rays, a two hour rest period following treatment and waiting in his office to be treated. The apparatus that was used for the treatment resembled a weight bench with a large drill press mounted at its head. The patient laid on the bench on either their right or left side. A stylus was lowered to the appropriate point on the neck and a switch triggered. In a fraction of a second the apparatus shot down against a predetermined point on the neck and applied over 100 pounds pressure to that spot in order to align the vertebrae. This happens in an instant and is more of a surprise than a discomfort. I laid down for the prescribed two hour period and went back to our trailer, my wife driving as required. The treatment seemed to help and I am still free of most of the "high neck" problems that I had been experiencing.

> **Cortisone cures nothing. It only relieves the symptoms of the condition being treated.**

42

Drugs! A Critical Decision

When I was still living in the area where I had my fusion performed, I went to the same doctor who had done my surgery for treatment of my neck problems. I knew he had run out of ideas when he suggested that he start treating me with regular injections of cortisone to help fight the pain.

Cortisone is a corticosteroid and is a hormone. It is secreted by the outer cover of the adrenal glands, which are located above the kidneys. It is used by the body as a protection against disease and shock.

Cortisone was discovered in 1935–36. Artificial cortisone was first produced ten years later. It is used in the treatment of numerous diseases. Cortisone cures **nothing**. It only relieves the symptoms of the condition being treated.

I spite of its attributes, cortisone also has many negative side effects. Some of these can be considered minor while others are more severe, even dangerous. Some of the side effects of cortisone consist of; falling blood pressure, mood changes, "moon face" a "buffalo hump" on the back, peptic ulcers, increased susceptibility to infections, osteoporosis, cataracts and psychological disturbances. In fact, after prolonged treatment, an abrupt withdrawal of the drug can cause death.

Now do you really wonder why I declined?

Many people with back and neck pain find that there are several exercises that strengthen the afflicted muscles and eventually relieve some of the discomfort. This seems to be especially true in cases of back pain. I had a man once tell me that if a person with back pain would spend about five minutes a day jumping softly on a miniature trampoline the resulting strengthening of the back muscles would alleviate most of their pain. This might be worth a try for someone with back problems. I have started more exercise programs than a fat man has diets. Invariably I end up pulling something in my neck, hurting for about two or three weeks and

43

then laying low for about six months before trying again. I have not given up on exercising, but I'm "off" more than "on."

You are going to have to deal with your pain predominantly at home. You are going to have to find some things that will help you in your battle against this untiring foe. I have tried several things over the years. Following is a list and description of what I have personally found helpful.

Hot Water

As mentioned earlier, soaking my neck in hot water tends to loosen the tight muscles and generally brings relief with it. It is the single most effective remedy that I personally have found. Also, as mentioned earlier, there is no possible way to do this when you live on the road in a travel trailer as we do.

Most of my preaching meetings start on Sunday and end on Friday. This makes Saturday our "driving day" in order to get to the next meeting. There are a few times when a meeting ends on Wednesday or Thursday because two days are needed to drive to the next meeting. In cases like this we generally stay overnight at a campground on our way to our destination. Sometimes in the winter we will spend a night in a motel rather than a campground just so that I can have access to a full size bathtub and plenty of hot water. Many times I have ended weeks of pain by a desperate visit to a motel for a soak in a tub.

Portable Heat

Since I cannot soak my neck on a regular basis, I do the next best thing. I lay my neck on something warm. I have found two excellent sources of this "portable heat."

The first is the common electric heating pad. I have spent many hours reading my Bible with a heating pad laid under the back of my neck. Although the heating pad helps, but isn't tremendously effective. I have noticed that the relief experienced by its use doesn't last very long once I get away from it. Still, in severe winters, which translates to "severe pain" for me, I have had to spend the better part of the day laying on a heating pad just so that I would be able to turn my head that night while preaching. Many times I have spent most of the day on a heating pad only to leave it just long enough to preach and then return to it as soon as the service is over.

My wife is truly a wonderful lady. She is always on the lookout for ways to help me both in the ministry and in life. One day she came into the trailer from shopping and handed me her greatest purchase. It looked like a sock that had been filled with sand and then had a handle sewed to each end. The instructions said that you were to put it in the microwave for three minutes. It would then radiate heat for about an hour. Sure enough, it worked! There are two obvious advantages that this microwave neck warmer has over the heating pad. The first is that it conforms to the shape of the neck better than the heating pad. This puts the heat closer to the problem. Secondly, if I have to go outside during the winter, I can wrap it around the back

> **I have never taken any vitamin or herb and then been able to notice a difference.**

of my neck and not only keep the cold away from my neck, but radiate heat into it even while outside.

Strangely, the heat from the neck warmer seems to have a longer lasting effect on my neck than does that of the heating pad. It is a "wet heat" which seems to penetrate better. It hasn't supplanted the heating pad entirely, but has taken an extremely important role along with it in my battle with pain.

"The Buffer"

Another of my constant companions in this never ending battle is "The Buffer." This device is really a two handed massager and is remarkably similar to an electric sander. Whenever I am "Froze Up" my wife usually works my neck and back over with "The Buffer." This tends to loosen up the muscles a little. I also use it on my head to help fight the pain from the headaches they accompany my condition. "The Buffer" has given me temporary relief that usually lasts long enough to accomplish some short term task.

Along this line is a fairly new device that works like two rotating fingers to massage the neck. This rotating finger movement helps to relax the muscles of a very stiff neck.

> **I have steadfastly refused to get any prescription pain killers for my pain. Why? Because they might work!**

When I first saw this device I was skeptical of its value. Then one day when my neck was "Froze Up" and a headache was threatening to take the top of my head off I tried one that a pastor friend had. The machine is flat enough to be able to lay flat and slip it under your head so that the rotating fingers can massage the neck muscles. The fingers can reverse direction at the flip of the power switch. One thing that I have learned over the years is that **nothing** acts fast. Whenever I hurt my neck by making a quick turn, I know that it will be hours before the real pain sets in. This is also true of anything that I use to combat pain. The relief is never instantaneous. I can use "The Buffer" or the rotating finger machine and I won't know if it has helped me until the next day. Well, the day after trying this rotating finger machine I was able to turn my head a little. Something that would have taken two or three days naturally. I had found another helper! I now own one.

Vitamins and Herbs

I am a believer in the value of including vitamin supplements in ones regular diet. I'm not a believer in the "everything we eat is poison" view of vitamins. But I do recognize their value in maintaining good health. I am not able though to trumpet their praise in the battle with pain.

I am always willing to try vitamins or herbs in my attempt to maintain my sanity. The sad fact is that it is almost impossible to tell if they are helping. I have never taken any vitamin or any herb and then been able to notice a difference. I do understand that, in many cases, they have to build up in your system in order to help. (Or at least this is a good "cover" argument used by their proponents.) But regardless, I have never been able to see any dramatic change from using them. Please understand, I take vitamin supplements everyday. But I take them for my general health as opposed to combating pain. (Please don't send me your suggestions.)

There is one thing about vitamins and herbs that I find almost unbearable. Their promoters! More than once I have been in absolute agony due to neck and head pain. Some vitamin popping genius will look at me like I am the stupidest thing on two legs and ask demandingly, "Do you take vitamins?" or "Have you rubbed tree bark on the bottom of your feet?" or, "Have you snorted frozen Dandelion root?" Then, before I can answer with, "What vitamins are you talking about?" they flippantly announce, "Take vitamin Z-28 and you'll never hurt again!" Having just educated another poor ignorant fool on how easy it is to get rid of pain, they confidently walk off. (Which does get rid of **one** pain in the neck!) It is good that they have left though, because when I am "under the influence" of extreme pain and then confronted by an arrogant "health expert" I tend to be a little short on patience. Their departure helps to keep me from saying, **or doing**, something that I may regret later in the privacy of a jail cell.

Aspirins and Pain Killers

Aspirins are the single most common type of pain killer that I allow myself. When a siege of pain hits that lasts for weeks I turn almost exclusively to aspirin. I am **not** indiscriminate about using them, though. I don't want to become dependent on **any** pill. Of course the continual use of aspirin over the years has done terrible things to the lining of my stomach. For this reason I am **very** careful about each aspirin that I take. The trick here is to be able to judge whether or not a slight head pain is "just passing through" or "coming to stay." If it is passing through it will soon leave without the need of an aspirin. If it is here to stay for awhile you need to "fire early" or it quickly develops into a three or four day affair that nothing seems to affect. (I have one of those now. I was late taking the aspirins and now its here for a few days.)

In an attempt to preserve my stomach lining I have tried taking coated aspirins. These are aspirins that are designed to pass through the stomach and then dissolve in the intestine thus, in theory, saving your stomach. The problem here is twofold. first, they seldom have any affect on my pain. Second, I figure that if an aspirin dissolving in the stomach damages the stomach lining, what does an aspirin dissolving in the intestine do to the lining of that organ? Scary thought!

I have tried most of the other commercially available pain killers with varying degrees of success. Tylenol doesn't even touch my pain. The others, such as Ibuprofin, work sporadically.

So far I have steadfastly refused to get any prescription pain killers for my pain. Why? **Because they might work!** I greatly fear becoming an indiscriminate user of prescription drugs. I know many people who have become addicted to prescription pain killers. It is all too easy to say "Well, I'll just be careful as to how I use them." But the problem is that you

48

don't think quite so rationally when you are experiencing a regular torture session with pain. It is just too easy to pop more pills, "Just this one time." The next thing you know, you're a junkie. I have not absolutely ruled out prescription pain killers. They may be looming somewhere in my future, but I have fought this pain for over twenty years and I intend to fight on until I have no other recourse but prescription drugs. I'm not there yet!

Call Me In the Morning

We have all heard accounts of people who have contacted a doctor by telephone with a problem only to be told to "Take two aspirins and call me in the morning." This is **not** a put off. A combination of aspirins and sleep is one of the best things you can do in fighting pain. Many of the times that I've taken a pain killer and had it not work was due to the fact that I took it and then immediately had to go out and teach or preach. If I had been able to take the pills and lay down and sleep for a couple of hours, they

> I noticed a tingling sensation down the length of my right arm. Soon I was having trouble gripping the steering wheel.

may have worked. In extreme cases I will take some aspirins, soak in a tub, "buff" my neck and then lay down and sleep for about two hours. The result is dramatic.

Most of my meetings run from Sunday through Friday. We have been known to drive up to sixteen hours on a driving day. If I dare get a headache during one of these trips I know that I am in for a **horrible** time. When this happens I will arrive at the church, set up the trailer, try to be cordial to the pastor and then beat a hasty retreat to the "The Buffer," aspirins and bed. On occasions where I've been unable to do this I have been physically sick from the pain and the expenditure of will power required to do my duty. Just as surely as sleep can be an enemy if I sleep wrong and hurt my neck. It can also be a great ally when I can get to sleep quickly after taking a few aspirins to combat pain.

Hypnosis

I have been advised by "experts" (**everyone** is an expert on pain relief) to try hypnotism to help deal with the pain. **I staunchly refuse!** In order to be hypnotized you must become passive and allow your will to be controlled by another party. This is an invitation to trouble. **Spiritual trouble!**

> **I was experiencing headaches that would last days and weeks.**

It is not that I fear that the person hypnotizing me may cause me to do something that I wouldn't do under other circumstances. It is that a person in a passive state (like watching television) is vulnerable to spirits that are not necessarily friendly to them. When you surrender control of yourself to someone else you can not be **sure** who will be **taking control** or how willing they will be to relinquish it again. Hypnosis is not to be considered in fighting pain or **any** of the problems of life.

Pressure Points

Once while at a meeting I heard a missionary's wife talking to someone about "pressure points" and how pain could be stopped by applying pressure to the proper places. At that time I was two days into horrendous head pain so I asked this lady to show my wife how to apply pressure in the proper manner. They laid me on my back on a table in a Sunday School room and applied pressure to two spots at the base of my skull. Though it was a little uncomfortable, it was far from unbearable. About an hour later the lady asked me how I felt. I told her that the pain in my head was subsiding, which it was. What I didn't tell her was that I had a slight sense of pain down the length of my right arm. I couldn't know if it would soon pass or not and didn't want to add a negative comment to what was obviously a positive help so I didn't mention it.

The next morning I left town on one of those rare occasions when I must leave my family and travel to a meeting alone. The drive would only be about four hours. The first thing that I noticed in the morning prior to leaving was that the pain in my right arm had definitely intensified. I said nothing to my wife. I don't like to continually weigh her down with reports of my pain. Once I got on the road the problems began to multiply. The pain in my arm became **intense**! I also noticed a tingling sensation down the length of my right arm also. Soon I was having a little trouble gripping the steering wheel with my right hand while the pain grew greater and greater. By the time I got to my destination I was in absolute agony concerning my right arm. I checked in with the pastor and then beat a retreat to the motel. During the next few days I "buffed" my neck and soaked it in the tub. I suffered through three more days of agony before the pain in my right arm subsided. I still experience numbness down my right forearm

> **Well-meaning or not, you wish that people would just leave you alone.**

and into my middle and ring fingers. I have sworn off pressure points. What does that mean? That means I will not allow anyone to use "pressure points" on me until some day in the future when I have been suffering with about a week of extreme pain in my head and I am then willing to trade the pain in my head for three or four days of pain and paralysis in my arm. There are no **simple solutions** when you live with pain.

"The Zapper"

At this time it has been twenty-three years since I broke my neck. I divide this time period into two parts, each one being eleven years in length and each with a **major crisis** at the end of the eleven year period. Each eleven year period also ended with an act of blessed intercession by God that saved my sanity.

The first crisis and its remedy has already been discussed. It was the problem that I had of experiencing deep and intense pain in my arms for long periods of time. When I knew that there was nothing that could be done to alleviate my problem, God allowed an indiscriminate tackle in a game of sandlot football to do what no doctor had been able to do in eleven years. My sanity was saved!

Eleven years after this event I was faced with another crises of sanity threatening proportions. This time the culprit was extreme and extensive periods of pain in my head. I was experiencing headaches that would last days and weeks of an intensity that bordered on mind numbing. The "Buffer," hot water and the heating pad were all to no avail. I was consuming **tons** of aspirins and my stomach was paying a severe price. My prayers were the same as they had been eleven years earlier. "Lord, I accept all of the pain that You want me to have, but I am at the point of breaking mentally from this and then I will be no good to anyone." As in the earlier case, I saw no hope of relief. It was shortly after this prayer and only about a month after starting this book that God sent His gracious help.

A short time after this I was preaching at a church in Cedar Rapids, Iowa when I was engaged in conversation with a brother in Christ who had suffered a neck injury similar to mine. He told me about the great amount of head pain he had been suffering with as a result of his injury. Obviously I understood his situation. Then he told me about a little device that he had made to counter the problem. It was nothing more than the electric spark igniter used on the common gas barbecue grill. It was a round black collar surrounding a red plunger. Press the red button and it produces a spark at the opposite end which is shaped similar to an automotive sparkplug. Around this igniter he had affixed two small pieces of plastic tubing. The top piece was about one and a half inches long and the bottom was one inch long respectively. These sections of tubing were separated by a thin piece of metal bent like the fingers of a syringe. You could hold the "Zapper" like a syringe, press it against the neck and depress the plunger with your thumb sending an electric charge into the skin. The entire device is only about four inches long.

The theory behind this device is that the electric charge is supposed to stimulate the nerves and allow more blood to reach the nerve endings, which in turn alleviates the pain. Whether this is what happens or not I do not know. What I **do know** is that it **greatly** reduced the pain in my neck. He had told me that in order to relieve the pain of a headache you were to "zap" the back of the neck, the webbing between the thumb and fore finger and the top side of the ankles. Sound crazy? Yes. Does it work? Yes! He gave me one. He had purchased the igniter at a hardware store for under ten dollars. I have used it extensively since that time. Here's what I have found. Like aspirin, I need to catch a headache before it can get settled in. If I do, I can usually head it off before it gets bad. If the headache gets established then I have to give it the full treatment of heat, aspirins, etc. Then I "zap" my neck like crazy and go to bed. The next day the headache is usually gone. What had been **weeks** of unbearable pain had been reduced to **a day** of unbearable pain. I cannot tell you what a great blessing that this is!

"The Zapper" is small enough to carry in your suit coat

pocket. (Though I don't think I'd try walking through an airport metal detector with it. It's not a weapon, but imagine yourself trying to explain to airport security what you claim it to be!) I have "zapped" myself while driving the car. I have "zapped" myself almost anywhere. I have even "zapped" myself while writing this book! I have experienced almost instantaneous relief to some degree. If this one goes bad I intend to make another as soon as possible. Once again. It was a simple little thing, like a football tackle, that has rescued my mind from the threat of insanity.

This causes me to wonder what my problem will be in eleven more years. But I like to think that the Lord will have returned by then and I will be in Heaven enjoying my new neck.

The Pain That Never Goes Away

Over the years, one of the most unavoidable pains has been the unsolicited advice of life's many experts. Some are arrogant idiots. Some are very well meaning people. Some are folks who just will never understand that all answers are not as simple as rubbing something on or popping a pill. No matter which, the endless recipes and suggestions wear my patience to the point of belligerence. I am cordial. I am polite. I generally nod my head and comment that "Yes, hanging upside down by the feet while suspended from the belly of an airplane flying at 10,000 feet could possibly relieve my pain." (So could a bullet to the brain but I don't intend on trying **that** either!) With all the pain that **cannot** be avoided, you find this brand maddening. Well meaning or not, you wish that people would just leave you alone.

5

Living With the Pain

There are several pitfalls of living with constant pain. The greatest of these is possibility that your mind will be so over-taxed by the constant assaults that you will simply go in-sane. This is no overstatement. Your mind can only handle a limited amount of input from nerve endings that are sound-ing a continual "pain alarm." Pain of any intensity that is unrelenting for several days or weeks can overload the mind's ability to handle the messages from the nerves. Then, like an overloaded electrical circuit, a "breaker" kicks. Simply put, you go insane. The pain becomes your only conscious thought and . . . **the battle is lost**.

I will present only one brief example. One will suffice to illustrate the pressure on the mind caused by continual, in-tense pain. Two would over stress the case and be a vehicle for pity rather than teaching.

A Week In a Life of Pain

This particular episode with pain is not out of the ordinary. Since I am preaching almost every night of the year except Saturday, the situation given is repeated many times during a year's time. Because I must fulfill my obligation to preach whether I am hurting or not there are the added pressures of "Press on regardless" and "Don't let them know." (I loath pity.)

The following is edited from the log I keep of meetings and happenings.

Monday

"I woke up with a headache. I took aspirins during the day and was able to keep the pain in check.

"Monday night as I preached, my head was splitting. After service I stood at the door and shook hands with people. Then we went back to the trailer. Kathy 'buffed' my neck and I took some more aspirins. Then we went into the pastor's house (where we were parked) for evening fellowship."

Tuesday

"The headache was gone when I woke up but it had been replaced with head **pain**. The battle continued most of the day but the pain never gained any ground. I victory for me!

"While I was preaching, the pain in my head intensified. Strobes of pain shot up the left side of my head. Once, while preaching, I moved wrong and gasped from a bolt of pain that shot down my neck. (I **hate** when I do that!) After preaching I endured the pain while I shook hands at the door. Then we hurried home and Kathy **again** 'buffed' my

> I closed the sermon, turned the service over to the pastor, and headed straight for his office.

head and neck for about twenty minutes. The skin on my neck was still tender from the previous night's 'buffing.' I took a few more aspirins and then 'zapped' my head and neck with 'The Zapper.' Then it was back into the pastor's house for fellowship."

---

[1] During this time I was studying for a television appearance where, along with two other men, I would face five scholars who disputed the perfection of the Bible. Pain is not a welcome "study partner."

Wednesday

"I woke up on this morning without pain in my head. But today's grief was numbness in my right forearm and hand.[1]

"As the day went on, pain began another assault on my head. I took some pain killers and went to church to preach. This was possibly the worst head pain that I have ever experienced while preaching. I came very close to stopping the sermon and apologizing and then leaving. It didn't help that this all took place during one of the hottest summers on record and the church had no air conditioning and only two small windows for ventilation.

"When I finished preaching I was in a near state of panic which I call, 'The Mexicans are coming over walls!' (i.e., The Alamo) This means that all of

> **It is during such sieges of pain that I dig my fingernails into 2 Corinthians 12:9.**

my defenses against the pain have crumbled and I am at the mercy of a merciless, ravaging enemy. I closed the sermon, turned the service over to the pastor, and headed straight for his office where I could be out of sight. There was no way possible for me to put on a smile and shake hands on this evening. I sat at his desk and writhed in pain until my wife came in. She knew that I was in trouble. We snuck out of the church and headed for our van. She drove, as I was in no shape to. My ten year old son stood behind my seat in the van on the way home and rubbed my head.

"When we arrived at the trailer she immediately gave me some aspirins and started 'buffing' my neck, back and head again. My skin was screaming from the irritation of a third consecutive night of 'buffing' but there was no other recourse. Following that treatment she rubbed on some liniment which I followed with more shocking of my neck and head with 'The Zapper.' I watched as 'the Mexicans' retreated back over the wall that had been so recently breached. I was safe for a while.

"By this time I was absolutely exhausted from the battle. I went straight to bed. There would be no fellowship this evening. The pastor, like so many others, understood the situation."

Thursday

"I woke up with a slight headache. My head felt like it was full of cotton. I started the day with another 'buffing' followed by another 'zapping' which was chased by a few more aspirins. Then I resumed my studying in preparation for an up coming television debate that I was scheduled to do.

"As soon as I started preaching my voice gave me trouble. When the doctor fused my vertebrae together back in 1973 my vocal cords contracted. It was four months before my voice returned. It has never been as strong as it had been and is now prone to give out on me without warning. Tonight it decided to give me trouble.

"I preached (screeched) my message anyway. About halfway through the message, pain again began to invade the left side of my head. It was not as bad as Tuesday and **not near** like Wednesday's attack.

"Following the service I was at my place at the door, shaking hands. Then it was back to the trailer for yet another 'buffing,' more 'zapping' and a couple more aspirins. That took care of it. Then into the pastor's house for fellowship."

Friday

"No pain! Just the weariness that comes from four long, hard days of battle."

It is during such sieges of pain that I dig my fingernails into 2 Corinthians 12:9; *"And he said unto me, My grace is sufficient for thee: for my strength is made perfect in weakness. Most gladly therefore will I rather glory in my infirmities, that the power of Christ may rest upon me."*

If I ever "break" it will be because I have ceased to believe this great promise and been washed away by the **hopelessness** that would accompany such a conclusion.

Yet Another Worry

Beside the fear of going insane, one of the greatest dangers that a person who lives with constant pain may fall victim to is that of becoming too self centered. This **is not** a self centeredness born of conceit or pride. Rather, it is caused by the fact that over a long period of time you slowly become a mental slave to your pain. You

> **There is a tendency through all of this to slowly drift into seclusion.**

give it too many concessions. Soon, your decisions are based only on what effect your actions may have your "condition." (I hate that word!)

This malady can manifest itself in several ways, none of which is helpful to you or anyone else around you.

Mental Selfishness

One way this problem may manifest itself is in the form of a fear of doing **anything**, least you hurt yourself and aggravate your misery. The sad fact is that this fear may be well justified. I know from my personal experience that I have accidentally hurt myself carrying out the most insignificant of tasks. An example is that, even though a football injury actually **helped** my condition, I quit playing football after that injury because I can't take the chance that the **next** injury may result in severe damage to my neck. I would **never forgive myself** if I exited the next football game on a stretcher, never to walk again. You may read this and try to figure out some way to minimize this fear, but then it isn't **your neck**!

Hurting yourself is never a sure thing. You may be able to enjoy an activity nine out of ten times without triggering a problem. But after a while, the suffering caused by that single instance so punishes you that you choose to do nothing rather than take a chance on provoking a "sleeping dog." Again, you may be **one hundred percent correct** in your action (or inaction) but it tends to take some of the joy out of living. You soon realize that not all handicaps are visible to the naked eye.

I can see no way to overcome this problem. Some conditions are simply very susceptible to being easily aggravated. Add to that the ceaseless onslaught of age and its corresponding complications and you have quite a **mental battle** to fight right along with having to contend with the pain itself. It is truly a never ending battle!

There is a tendency through all of this to slowly drift into seclusion. Personally I think that pain is a private thing. I do not wish to sit around and discuss my pain with the people around me. Writing a book about it is one thing, but being forced to discuss it with each new person that I meet is I fate I would find unbearable. I don't even tell my wife about the running battles that I fight with pain. I only bother her when I must enlist her help for the fight. For this reason, when I am experiencing extreme pain, I try to remove myself from those around me. Being a preacher, which is without a doubt one of the most **public** of life-styles, makes it somewhat difficult if not impossible to withdraw yourself from a crowd. This is especially true when many individuals among them have been waiting for an opportunity to speak

> **You mentally see only your own pain and ignore or downplay the problems of others. Anybody can get tired of a constant complainer.**

with you. As you saw earlier, I generally try to fulfill what I consider my ministerial obligations to people in spite of any discomfort that I might be experiencing at that particular time. There are times though that I consider myself "no good to anyone" because of the overbearing effects of exceptionally extreme pain. At times like this I try to circulate among the crowd briefly following the service and then disappear from sight. I don't like to do this, but you can only endure so much pain before your ability to concentrate on others is impaired.

The problem that arises from this is that the welcome relief from the pressure (not the pain) that comes with being alone may become too inviting. You may find yourself exiting a scene when you really aren't hurting bad enough to justify it. I try to monitor my motives and to inventory my individual complications to assure myself that I'm not just "coping out." Too much seclusion is bad for the mind. But when "The Mexicans are coming over wall!" there is nothing you can do but "cut and run."

An even worse result of long term pain is that you mentally see only your own pain and ignore or downplay the problems of others.

There are **many** people who suffer from serious and genuine pain of their own or who are going through a crisis of some sort. When you are constantly concentrating on controlling your own pain so that you can mingle in a crowd without screaming at the top of your lungs you have less mental effort to sympathize or offer help to someone who comes to you with a genuine problem. This is not to mention the person who only **thinks** they have a problem or who simply wants to monopolize your time.

Some times your disinterest is not a problem of a cold heart. An individual can mentally support only a limited amount of thought processes at one time. When you are mentally, and secretly, involved in directing your own actions in spite of pain you simply cannot concentrate well on the problems of others. This greatly inhibits your ability to help people and leads you only deeper into self centeredness and seclusion.

My wife is a **tremendous** lady. She is a Christian who has always put the Lord first in her life. She is a wonderful mother to our children and she is a fantastic wife to me. Over the twenty-three years that we've been married she has been an extraordinary helpmate to me. She not only helps me in the areas where I ask her to but she also looks for things that she can do for me on her own. She would be this kind of a person even if I had never broken my neck. Yet to this exceptional wifely performance she has had to endure the additional burden of her husband being in pain most of his waking hours. Here too she has been exemplary. She is always looking for things that may help me combat my pain. She is the one who found the microwave neck warmer and bought it for me. She has spent hours "buffing" my neck with "The Buffer" trying to loosen my muscles and relieve some of my pain. She ever feels only sympathy for my plight and has **never** shown signs of "getting tired of it." She never complains about my complaining!

> You may wear out the compassion of a spouse who does love you and really wants to help.

There are two important things I keep in mind concerning my wife. The first is that, even though she has always been understanding towards my pain, **anybody** can get tired of a constant complainer. I would like to think that I "suffer in silence" as much as possible concerning my pain. Even though the fact is that I really do keep pretty quiet about the lower, more common end of the spectrum of pain; "the stone in my shoe', "the Pit Bull," "the Ax," I am too much of a weakly to bear the more intense, longer duration pain in silence. Right or wrong, when you move your head and pain shoots through your neck, **you gasp**. In spite of all this, my wife has **never** looked down on me. Yet you must be ever conscience not to complain about **ever pain**, **every day**. Be careful not to constantly complain. You may wear out the compassion of a spouse who does love you and really wants to help but does not need to hear about every little ache that you have.

There is also a great truth that must not be ignored. Sometimes **your spouse** is going to be in pain and need **your help and understanding**. Over these twenty-three years there have been times when my wife has been injured in some way. There have been deaths in her family or problems with others which broke her heart and brought weeping to her soul. There have been two separate surgeries on her ears in an effort to prevent deafness from a disease that she has. (She wears two hearing aids.) There has been the recovery needed from delivering each of our three sons following difficult births. Our first son weighed ten pounds and two ounces. During the times when your spouse is hurting, either emotionally or physically, it is extremely important that you put your own discomfort aside and minister to the needs of the one you love. You **cannot** allow sympathy, patience and physical care to apply only to

> **During the times when your spouse is hurting, either emotionally or physically, it is extremely important that you put your own discomfort aside and minister to the needs of the one you love.**

you. You **must be there** for the one you love, **regardless of your own problems**! Don't be self-centered!

It also would not hurt your situation to take your spouse out to dinner to show them that you appreciate what they do for you in your personal battle with pain. Such actions let them know that you are not ignorant of the many sacrifices and service that they experience on your behalf.

Another dangerous pitfall of constant pain is that of becoming a "mental cripple." After a while you begin to feel that no one cares or **cares enough** about your problem. You find yourself angry when any attention is turned toward the pain or problems of someone else, to the exclusion of your own. After all, you are **obviously** in more need of help than **they** are. When you reach this point you are just about useless. You are like anyone who is on welfare who gets plenty of help but is angry at not getting **all of the help**. You will also exclude yourself from any requirements to help others or to serve the Lord. You have simply resigned yourself to being a spiritual welfare case. Soon you will be complaining about your ill treatment by others to anyone who will listen, and your audience will decrease with time since no one can stand being around someone who constantly complains. This only adds to your insolation and your feeling of rejection. No matter how bad you feel, **you can not see only your own problems and ignore the legitimate needs of others**. Too many "invalids" are volunteers. They reason that, "If you're crippled no one expects too much of you." It sure beats workin'! But there is a kind of "death in the pot" that will alter your personal outlook on life to the point of making you a social outcast. Physical pain is more than enough

> **You cannot allow sympathy, patience and physical care to apply only to you.**

to have to live with. Don't make yourself repulsive to others by your continual harping.

Sympathy—A Poor Substitute for Respect

Many a young man, in "love" with a girl who is no longer interested in him, has found that he can rekindle her interest in him by garnering her sympathy. He simply has to "get hurt" and she feels sorry for him and just can't bring herself to "abandon" him in his "hour of need." Some men have even managed to secure a

> **Sympathy prior to marriage becomes disrespect after marriage.**

wife this way. The problems with this tactic begin to arise after the marriage. Through years of counseling I have learned this truth about sympathy; **"Sympathy prior to marriage becomes disrespect after marriage."** In other words, that which turns her heart before marriage turns her stomach after it!

The reason for this is simple. **Before** marriage two individuals are unattached. The young man's "pain" has no influence over the young lady's life. She sees him as someone who needs pity and willingly supplies it.

After marriage her view changes. Now she sees her "wage earner" finding seemly insignificant reasons for why he can't work or pull his own weight around the house. It doesn't take long before her big brave "wounded soldier" is instead looked at as a sniveling cry baby who's first and final escape from all responsibility is, "I'm not feeling good today." Neither of them may be conscious of it, but her sympathy for her husband is evaporating and it is being replaced by disrespect for what she sees as a big "Cry Baby." Someone who is never lacking an excuse as to why he can't work or do anything.

Everyone enjoys the attention that comes from having a slight injury. There is what I call the "Million Dollar Injury." That is when you have been hurt bad enough to need sympathy but not bad enough to have to go to the hospital for treatment of your injury. "No. Just let me rest this old knee here while you make me a cup of coffee and get the evening newspaper for me and I should be all right in a few days . . . or weeks." You may be able to "bag 'em" with sympathy, but you can't "keep 'em."

When you have chronic pain it can become too easy to seek sympathy rather than face the responsibilities of life. I am a husband and a father. I have obligations to my wife and children and "hurting" is no acceptable excuse for not fulfilling those duties. I have three sons and I still take time out to wrestle with them. I cannot count the number of times I have hurt my neck doing this, but it is necessary when raising children. It would be easy to say, "I can't do that because of my neck" and then kick back and read a book.

> When you have chronic pain it can become too easy to seek sympathy rather than face the responsibilities of life.

There are enough activities that I simply cannot partake of with my sons (like football!). I don't need to cut off every form of physical activity. If you have a problem that gives you considerable pain or impairment you need to be careful not to shirk the responsibilities you have to those around you. Whether you are a husband or a wife, A father or a mother, there are things that are your exclusive responsibility around your home. It may be home repairs or it may be cooking. It may be discipline or it may be dialogue. You cannot let your pain reduce you to being nothing more than a **spectator** as life goes by and your family grows up. You must force yourself into activity.

Added to this problem is the guilt that you unconsciously feel from not performing tasks that you know that you are capable of. You will tend to overstate the case for your pain in an effort to convince yourself and others that you are not shirking your responsibilities. But, even if those around you accept your excuse, you will know down deep inside that you are just a charlatan who is using a legitimate problem for an illegitimate purpose. Come on! Toughen up! Do what you know you should when you know you can!

Another problem with sympathy is that your friends will soon tire of having to "baby sit" you every time that you are around. No one likes to be around a grown up who acts like a baby. Your friends and family, like anyone else, want to be with "normal" people. Therefore, you need to be as "normal" as possible. Think about it. You may think that walking with a limp

> **People eventually tire of always having to deal out special treatment.**

is great for garnering sympathy. But when you see someone else walking with a limp do you feel sympathy for them or gratitude that you can walk correctly? **Normal** is the best situation. We would all be better off if we had no problems to disrupt the normal performance of our assigned tasks. But in those situations where we do have problems, they need to be restricted from having anymore affect on our lives than absolutely necessary.

You may have some great fantasies about people feeling sorry for you in your "condition," but the fact is that people eventually tire of always having to deal out special treatment to some one else. And that won't be changed by **any amount** of "handicapped" legislation that Congress may pass.

Every person in this world can be classified as either a producer or a consumer. You either **give** or you **take**. It is essential that you don't drift into the "taking" segment of society and use your pain as an excuse to do so. There are enough legitimate causes of failure in life without always falling back on "pain" as an excuse for doing nothing. You should see to it that you pull your own weight in life.

I am fortunate that what I do does not require a great deal of physical strength. Over the years and after numerous trips to many doctors I am officially listed as 65% handicapped. I quit going to the doctor simply because I couldn't live with seeing that percentage slip closer to 100%. Although there are no outward signs to suggest a problem, I can thank God that I am not required to exert any great amount of physical strength. Conversely, I attempt to contribute more than what is normally associated with the ministry. I have been at meetings where I have painted the church doors or a new church sign or even the pastor's car. Why? Because it is easy enough for an **evangelist** to be a "taker." It is even easier for an evangelist with a broken neck to sit back and do nothing. I want to be a "giver." I want to **contribute** to the lives of those with whom I come in contact. I don't want to be a continual recipient of sympathy and special treatment.

> **Pick up some "shrink book" on how to "cope" with your problem and you're doomed!**

There are times when just doing your duty is trying. I have preached when I couldn't move my head. More times than can be counted I have preached with a monstrous headache. I have found something out about headaches. If I have a regular headache and preach anyway, the headache is usually gone by the time that I get done preaching. If I have a headache caused by my neck being "out," I am no better and sometimes worse after a service. It never matters though. You preach! Because that is what you're there for. I am not at a church so people can pity me and do special favors for me. **I am not there to "get"!** I am there to **GIVE!**

From "Cop Out" to "Cope Out"

Whatever your duties are, you will **never** find satisfaction by successfully shirking them. The less that you do, the worse you will feel. The worse that you feel, the less you will do. Now all you need to do is pick up some "shrink book" on how to "cope" with your problem and you're doomed! You don't need to sit around and wallow in your pain. Many of the books offered by today's psychologists offer no more help for hurting people

> **My pain is not a "thorn in the flesh"! It is a pain in the neck!**

than to give them an excuse for doing nothing. Today there are millions of people who have been made "mental cripples" by "discovering" that they were "sick" because of something that they read among the ramblings of a fantasying "expert." They use what they have read as a licence to do nothing and as proof of the need for sympathy and preferential treatment. **Burn** the "shrink" books, **Read** your Bible and **get to work!**

You need to get out and find something to do that will be a help to others. You will never feel better than when you have done something for someone else.

What It Isn't!

People who live with continual pain of some sort are as familiar with what the Bible says about having a "thorn in the flesh" as any mission bum is with the scripture that says, *". . . use a little wine for thy stomach's sake. . . ."* Talk with an old wino for any length of time and someplace in the conversation he will quote this fraction of 1 Timothy 5:23. The **worst part** about it is that he will self righteously act as though he is a Bible scholar when it comes to the subject of drinking. Apparently, since he spends so much of his waking hours drinking himself blurry he thinks that he is somehow an expert on this particular portion of scripture.

People who suffer from constant pain are the same way with 2 Corinthians 12:7 which reads; *"And lest I should be exalted above measure through the abundance of the revelations, there was given to me a thorn in the flesh, the messenger of Satan to buffet me, lest I should be exalted above measure."*

> ## You are above your pain in importance.

I don't know how many times I've had someone tell me about a physical problem and end their story by casually saying, "Well, Paul had his thorn in the flesh and I guess I've got mine!" The worst part about this is that they quote the passage just like the wino quotes First Timothy. They say it as though having some physical pain makes them a more spiritual person in some way.

Baloney!

Remember this. Paul had actually been in Heaven. He had seen and heard things that no living man ever had. The Bible says that God gave him a "thorn in the flesh" because he was in danger of being so spiritual that he might be "exalted above measure." I really don't believe that you or I are in danger of being **that** spiritual!

People love to get **spiritual** credit for a **physical** problem. There are Christians who don't tithe, don't attend church regularly, don't read their Bible, never win a soul to Christ and are generally about as spiritual as a rock. Yet, because they honestly suffer from some sort of physical pain they like to claim that it is their "thorn in the flesh" and that it has somehow made them closer to God than those who serve Him faithfully but don't suffer a physical problem.

My pain **IS NOT** a "thorn in the flesh"! It is **A PAIN IN THE NECK!** Hurting does not qualify me for some special Bible insight. It makes me no more an expert on 2 Corinthians than being a drunk makes someone an expert on 1 Timothy.

> **Slavery is still slavery. Whether you serve another man or yourself.**

I read thirty pages of my Bible everyday. I spend hours in prayer. I endeavor to ferret out my sins and personality problems so that I will be a better Christian. **THAT** is how you get close to God. Not by suffering from a physical problem yet doing nothing for the Lord Jesus Christ. Your pain does not make you spiritual. It makes you hurt!

Call it what it is. But don't call it what it isn't.

Push Yourself

You will never know what you can do in spite of your pain until you push yourself. There are many things that you are capable of, but they are not getting done because you have already told yourself that they are outside of your ability to perform them.

Let me give you a personal example. I had always restricted myself to writing no more than one book at a time. I just couldn't bring myself to concentrate on writing two books concurrently. I couldn't even bring myself to **start** a second book until the previous one I was working on was finished with type setting, printing and shipping. Duties that are not mine to do. When I had the new book "in hand" I then felt enough mental release to start writing another one.

This is how I did things for several years. Then we endured some severe attacks by the devil. These were not all related to the problems with my neck. It made me mad! As a form of a counter attack I determined that I would commence work on multiple books at the same time. I started three different books. Ironically, during the time I've been working on these three different projects, I sat down and started a fourth, **this book**. I now regularly work on several books concurrently. There was a time when I would never have believed that I could do that. Then I "pushed" myself.

Push **yourself!** See what you can do for the Lord that you have been claiming that you couldn't do because of your "condition." Pain or no pain, get active for the Lord. You won't get anything done barricading yourself in your home feeling sorry for yourself.

You're #1

This is not an attempt to psyche you into thinking that you possess more value than you really do. I am **not** into the present "self worth" scam that seems to be sweeping Bible believing Christianity. This is not a book on self worth. It is a book on self **ability**. When I refer to "you" as "#1," I mean that you are **above your pain** in importance. **"You" are not your body!** You are the soul that resides **inside of your body**. Your pain is limited to your flesh. You may do some things to curtail or suppress your pain. But if you ever let it run your life you are ruined.

An alcoholic is a **soul** that is a **slave to a body**. He says "I (the Soul) don't want to take a drink. But I (the Body) need it." His body is addicted to liquor and his soul can't say "No!" to his body. **Every** addiction is like this. Whether it is an addiction to drugs, sex, rock music, phobias or anything else. An addiction is simply a soul who has less will power than its body.

In the case of pain, you don't become **addicted** to it. You just become a **slave** to it. Sometimes your body can get out of hand. You will find it giving you problems just because there is something going on that it doesn't like. This is exactly what happens when a child, forced to eat something that he doesn't like, throws up. His body actually threw a

72

"tantrum." Now he will refuse to eat that particular food again because he thinks that it makes him sick. He is becoming a slave to his body.

This is why you should not be "religious" in catering to your pain. The most effective things that I do to relieve pain are heat, "The Buffer," "The Zapper," pain killers and sleep. Yet there are times **I absolutely refuse** to go through "the ritual" to fight my pain. I refuse to do things that will please my body even if it means that I may have to suffer for it. (See what I mean by the "battle" with pain?) Either I am going to serve **my body**, or **my body** is going to serve **me**. I have chosen the latter! Slavery is still slavery. Whether you serve another man or yourself.

You must not allow yourself to be bullied by your flesh until it makes you a "pain-oholic," unable to say "No" to anything that your body demands. Mind you. I'm not foolish. When the pain is so bad that I literally cannot see straight I do whatever I must to relieve it. But I also make sure that I do some things that my body doesn't approve of just to let it know who is in **overall** control in my life.

You should be reasonable in taking care not to aggravate your problem with pain. But you must also have enough will power not to become a slave to your body.

6

Help That No Doctor Can Give

Medical doctors are a blessing. Although they rank right up there with lawyers and politicians when it comes to the public's opinion of them, they are a great help to those in need. If you have ever needed serious medical help, you can probably thank a medical doctor for helping to restore you to good health. No matter **what** he charged you!

Most people are not aware that it is necessary for medical students to take out literally **thousands** of dollars in loans in order to complete their education. Graduation is followed by thankless years as an intern working under conditions that are not always the best. Added to this is the extreme pressure of continual testing which, if not passed, can prohibit them from ever practicing medicine. If that was not enough pressure, now our socialist minded government wants to socialize medicine. This will destroy our medical system. (Although the politicians that pass the law will have access to **private** medicine.)

> **There is help and hope to be accessed in the Bible that no medical doctor can offer.**

As a rule, people like to complain, and medical doctors are a favorite target. **Believe me!** I understand about both the dangers and irresponsibility of a doctor who overlooks a patient's injury. But we should also be thankful both for the great medical system that our nation has and for those who have given their lives to help people in need. Sure they get paid for it. You get paid for your labors. Don't you?

> **Ignore the needs of your soul and you are in great danger.**

In all of this, though, there are absolute limits to what a medical doctor can do for a patient. Their practice is limited to the physical. Although there are some who may tinker with the mind of their patients through the use of psychology, they are not able to minister to the **spiritual** side of a patient. Yet we Christians are able to enlist help from both the **spiritual** as well as the physical. We have direct access to God through prayer and from God through His word, the Bible. I can **assure you by the authority of the Bible** that there is help and hope to be accessed in the Bible that no medical doctor can offer.

There are two things you can **and should** do if you are plagued by continual pain.

Feed Your Soul

You feed your flesh physically by eating, thus giving yourself the physical strength to carry out the duties of life.

You feed your mind and emotions by doing what you must to relieve the discomfort brought on by pain. This is how you protect yourself from the mental stress brought on by daily bouts with pain.

It is therefore **imperative** then that you also **feed your soul**. Ignore the needs of your soul and you are in great danger.

There is only one way to strengthen your soul in order to strengthen it against your flesh. You must "feed" your body the Bible. There are two ways to do this. Listen carefully! **If you count this portion of this book as unimportant you have missed it all**. This is the singly most important part of this book. If you are going to ignore this advice then just throw this book away, throw your Bible away and then keep taking drugs until you no longer know what day of the week it is, because you have **surrendered the battle**.

You get spiritual input from the Bible in two ways. The first is through church attendance. You need to sit yourself down in front of a preacher and let him skin you alive! Your flesh is wicked (Jeremiah 17:9) and the more preaching that you subject your body to, the better chance you have of gaining some control over it. God chose the "foolishness" of preaching by which to save the lost. (1 Cor. 1:21) Preaching is the single greatest deterrent to allowing your flesh to run (ruin!) your life.

You may get upset by the preaching that you hear. But it is good for you to learn to endure it and then later to apply it to your life. I am by no stretch of the imagination referring to the socialist whining that is passed of as preaching from the modernist pulpits across America. I am referring to attendance at a fundamental, Bible believing, independent Baptist church. Your prejudice, or that which has been

> **Opening the Bible and reading it exposes you to something spiritual that no book on "coping" ever will.**

superimposed on you by the media, may reject this prescription. But let's face the facts. How many times have you had to take some medication or submit to surgery that you **also** rejected, but needed? Get to church!

The other way that you feed your soul is by reading your Bible on a daily basis. I have always recommended that people should read a Proverb each day, to correspond with the day's date. That will put you through the entire Book of Proverbs in a month. That will put you through the entire Book of Proverbs (and put the Book of Proverbs **through you!**) twelve times in a year.

The Book of Psalms speaks to the **spirit**. That's why so many people run to it when they are troubled and need their **spirit** uplifted. But the Book of Proverbs speaks to your **soul**. You will never read a proverb but that you will see something lacking in your personality. You will see things that you can do to make yourself a better person as well as help you endure your pain.

> I simply lay myself before the Lord and ask Him to listen to the "groanings" which I cannot utter.

Along with reading a Proverb for the corresponding calendar date I also **strongly urge** people to read ten pages of the Bible **everyday**. You should begin at Genesis and read to the end of Revelation. Then you should start all over and do it again. Then you should do it again. You should keep reading your Bible cover-to-cover on a daily basis until you **die** or until you hear **a real loud trumpet!** Reading ten pages per day will put you through the entire Bible three to three and a half times each year. You cannot believe the help that daily Bible reading will be in your battle with pain. Not only are there verses that may apply to your situation, but simply being exposed to God's Book will help you. You may claim that ten pages per day is too much. It is not! If you read other books, I am sure that you have sat down and read thirty or forty or perhaps fifty pages at a sitting. You have probably gone to bed much later than you planned on. What was your excuse? "I just couldn't put it down!" If you can read that many pages of an **uninspired** book, then ten pages of the Bible is not unreasonable.

> If you give up on God's word, why shouldn't He give up on you?

Nutritionists say that they cannot trace how protein gets from the food you eat to each cell in your body. Neither can I explain exactly how the Bible helps you. But daily Bible reading will strengthen you (the Soul) against your flesh (the Body). You may not remember what you read. You may not entirely understand what you read. But simply opening the Bible and reading it exposes you to something spiritual that **no book on "coping" ever will**. I cannot over stress the need to read your Bible on a daily basis. Your soul (YOU) is spiritual and there is **nothing** that can feed a soul the spiritual nutrients that it needs but the Bible. **NOTHING!** As I said before, if you are not going to read your Bible then you may just as well take dope until your brain turns to jelly, because there is nothing that can do for you what the Bible can. You can neglect your physical needs a little bit in your battle with pain, but you dare not ignore the spiritual. **There is no substitute for Scripture!**

I have alluded several times in this book to the danger of going insane from the suffering brought on by continual pain. **Only the Bible** can assure you that this won't happen. As I quoted earlier, 2 Corinthians 12:9 declares, *"And he said unto me, My grace is sufficient for thee: for my strength is made perfect in weakness. Most gladly therefore will I rather glory in my infirmities, that the power of Christ may rest upon me."* It is impossible for me to count how many times I have turned to the truth of this scripture when I felt that I simply could bear no more pain. The Bible is

always right! If you feel like you can't stand anymore pain and the Bible says that you can, then I can assure you that **you can**. Again, this **is not** "the power of positive thinking." It is rather the assurance of your Creator that **His grace** can get you through **your pain**.

There is **never** a day when I am not in pain. I am constantly cracking my neck in hopes of getting some small amount of relief. There are also the "Black Days" when it takes all the will power that I have just to function. I have long ceased praying for a cessation of the pain since it is obvious at this point that that simply is not the will of God. But I do plead with God on those days when I feel like sanity is a granite wall and I am holding on by my fingernails. Many times I cannot frame the words of grief and so I simply turn to the truth assured us in Romans 8:26 which says, *"Likewise the Spirit also helpeth our infirmities: for we know not what we should pray for as we ought: but the Spirit itself maketh intercession for us with groanings which cannot be uttered."*

On such days I simply lay myself before the Lord and ask Him to listen to the "groanings" which I cannot utter. Do you have any idea of the peace and reassurance that comes from **knowing** that your prayers are getting through to God **exactly** how you need them to and that there

> **Do you have any idea what help you have when people are approaching God's throne everyday and interceding for you?**

can be no misunderstanding? **God is on our side!** If you abandon His Book, you abandon His help! No books, **including this one**, can do for you what the Bible can.

You don't need "mind over matter" books. You don't need

to learn how to "cope" with your situation. A psychologist, whether he is **lost or saved**, can only feed you the warmed over theories of Christ rejecting men who are determined not to submit themselves to God. **Is that what you need?** NO!

You need to read broken hearted David and commune with the same God that he communed with. You need to read Job. Not to compare your plight to his but to see that **God did deliver him**! You need the tender reassurance that God gives you in 1 Corinthians 10:13 when He had Paul write, *"There hath no temptation taken you but such as is common to man: but God is faithful, who will not suffer you to be tempted above that ye are able; but will with the temptation also make a way to escape, that ye may be able to bear it."*

You need the assurance Isaiah gives us when states in Isaiah 26:3, *"Thou wilt keep him in perfect peace, whose mind is stayed on thee: because he trusteth in thee."* Or what he says in chapter 41, verse 10, *"Fear thou not; for I am with thee: be not dismayed; for I am thy God: I will strengthen thee; yea, I will help thee; yea, I will uphold thee with the right hand of my righteousness."*

You will need the instruction of Lamentations 3:26–27, or the solemn warning of Proverbs 24:10. I could go on and on. There are literally **countless** verses that God can use to minister to your spiritual and emotional needs. But the Bible is useless if you can find an excuse for not reading it. But if you will read it, it will give you help from a source that is literally **out of this world**!

> **No dollar can relieve pain like prayer can.**

Now tell me! Can "Doctor Feelgood" do for you what old King James can? No. Never! Dump the "shrink" books. Dump your "modern version." Now sit down and bury your nose and your heart . . . **and your troubles** between the covers of the Bible that God has used for centuries. The King James Bible! A great man once said, "The Bible doesn't need to be **rewritten**. It needs to be **reread**!"

You don't need men's theories, opinions or outright chicanery. Theories change with time. Men make mistakes. Men **lie**! God does none of these. He is **always right. Always dependable**. Why would you abandon the Creator when the problem you have is with the creation that He made? If He made it, shouldn't He know how best to take care of it? "Healing lines" are great for securing new Cadillacs for the preacher supposedly doing the healing. But all you need is to open the pages of God's

> **You should get yourself addicted to prayer.**

divine Book and bask in its radiance. "Coping" isn't the answer. Maybe even "curing" isn't the answer. But getting in touch personally with God through His Book will help you more than anything and everything that man has to offer.

If you give up on God's word. Why shouldn't He give up on you?

Get Addicted to Prayer

Mr. Webster says that to be addicted to something you must "devote or surrender yourself to something habitually." **That** is what you need to do with prayer.

If you suffer from continual pain you should do all that you can to get God's people praying for you. One of the benefits of traveling all over the country and being in a different church every week is that I get to meet thousands of born-again, Bible believing, God loving Christians. Quite frequently someone will ask me, "What can I do for you?" This usually means, "Do you need some money?" Although money may be nice to receive, no amount of money can replace the power of a Godly Christian praying for you. I usually answer, "When you think off me, **pray for me**." Whenever I am asked by someone if there is something in particular that I would like them to pray for I ask them to pray for my neck. No details. Just, "Pray for my neck."

There are hundreds, if not thousands, of Christians who pray for my neck. I will often walk into a church that I haven't been in for years and have someone walk up and say, "I pray for you everyday!" Do you have any idea what help you have when people are approaching God's throne **everyday** and interceding for you?

Evangelists are sometimes ulterior about getting people to give them money or gifts. They will often try to endear themselves to someone in a church that they think that they can get some sort of financial help from. I am that way about prayer.

Listen! You can **always** get a dollar somewhere. They all look alike and they are gone faster than you desire. But prayer! Each individual's prayer, is

> **You must give prayer as well as receive.**

just that. An individual, independently imploring God to ease your pain. Why would I try for a dollar when I can get so much more help through the individual, loving prayers of God's people? No dollar can relieve pain like prayer can.

You should ask your church to remember to pray for your pain. (Not every week. Don't **be** a pain!) Certainly, some will forget to pray for you. But **someone** will remember your need and speak with God about it on your behalf. That's **ONE**! Ask your Christian friends and family to remember you in prayer. Get everyone praying for you that you can. (But **don't** be a "Nag.")

I take about forty-eight week long revival meetings per year. My meetings usually start Sunday and run through Friday. Then on Saturday we will hook our trailer to our van and drive for 8–12 hours to the next meeting. We will drop the trailer and set it up and do the same thing all over again on the next Saturday.

This tends to be a grueling pace. Add to that the fact that I also spend my time writing books, publicly debating the authority of the Bible and flying out of the country to preach a revival meeting or teach national pastors on the history of the Bible.

If everything in my life was exactly as it is now, except that there was **no one** praying for me, I could not do this. I could not continue on without the prayers of caring Christians. You see. **I am addicted to prayer**.

You should get yourself addicted to prayer. You will gain help that would be totally inaccessible in any other manner.

Don't Be Selfish

Don't forget! You are not the only person in the world suffering some kind of pain. Therefore you are not the only person in the world that needs prayer. Prayer is as easy to give as it is to get. You should have several people who suffer some kind of pain that you pray for regularly.

> **Kind words and dinner for two speaks volumes.**

I keep an "Everyday Prayer List" in my Bible at the day's Proverb. That way, I must see it everyday. I pray for these people before I read my Proverb. That way I can be sure that I will pray for them every single day.

I also pray for the physical problems of others, both friends and acquaintances.

I met a man in a church in Toledo, Ohio that endures neck pain similar to mine. I often remember to ask God to ease his suffering.

I have a friend who had Polio when he was a child and

has been on crutches most of his life. Several years ago I read that many people who had Polio in their youth are experiencing relapses that are leaving them bedridden. I pray frequently that God will spare my friend from this fate.

I know a man who has been in a wheelchair since being wounded while serving in the military in Vietnam. I pray for his physical problems often.

Then, there will be the stranger that I see hobbling down the road on crutches or in a wheelchair. I ask God to relieve their discomfort also. There are many others.

You must **give** prayer as well as **receive** it. You must be careful not to forget that you are not the only person in the world with a problem. Nor are you the most important person in the world. You are just one insignificant person with a problem that most of the world knows or cares nothing about. You have a problem that many others who are worse off than you are would love to be afflicted with, instead of what they have. Don't abandon others and then expect everyone to pray for you. Give. Give. Give. You will get plenty.

If you ignore the spiritual help offered through the Bible and personal prayer, you are not serious about getting relief from your pain for you have deserted the two primary sources of help that God has provided for you. Get help! Get reading! Get praying!

A Good Marriage Helps

A marriage in which the husband and wife are constantly at each other's throat is a grief. If you add to such a situation the mental stress of being in constant pain it can fast become unbearable. Therefore you should make it a point to make your marriage as good as you possibly can.

My wife and I have been hopelessly in love since we met. We love each other's company. We love the ministry that God has placed us in. We love and enjoy the children that the Lord has given us. The Lord has truly blessed us with a happy life.

The marriage relationship that Kathy and I share goes a **long way** in helping me to bear the pain that I experience. I may have to put up with the physical pain of a broken neck. But, **Praise the Lord!** I don't have to suffer the emotional pain of a broken heart.

Physical pain is something that you can't avoid, but marital pain can be avoided.

If you suffer from chronic pain you should work hard to make your marriage a good one. You should do what you can to make your spouse happy. I **am not** implying that a man should forfeit his manhood and become "hen pecked" just to assure peace in the family. Neither am I saying that a woman should be a mindless slave. I am simply stating that you should be affectionate a gracious to your spouse.

My wife is a tremendous wife and mother. She loves her household duties as well as the added responsibility of schooling our boys. I cannot express how much I appreciate her gracious ways! Therefore, I make a point of being kind to her. I try to be extra understanding to her griefs. I look for little things that I can get for her. She pleases me so very greatly in her actions toward me. Therefore I try to be pleasing in my actions toward her.

You need not humiliate yourself or spend vast amounts of money to show your appreciation to your spouse. Kind words and dinner for two speaks volumes. Remember. Deal with what you **can** have a positive influence on (your marriage) when you are saddled with something that you **cannot** have a positive influence on (your pain).

7

You Ain't Seen Nothin' Yet

Life with constant and/or intense pain is miserable. You never feel completely "good." You always find yourself restricted in what you are able to do. As if that was not bad enough, there are those occasions when you feel that you will go insane from the never ending assault that the pain makes on your mind. There tends to be a hopelessness to life. Yet, as bad as our physical pains and discomforts can be. There is something **far worse**. And **this** is a grief that you can avoid!

"A Bad Day Fishing . . ."

We've all seen the bumper sticker that says, "A Bad Day Fishing Is Better Than A Good Day Working!" Whether this is true or not, I'm not sure. But I do know this; **"A Bad Day Living With Pain Is Better Than A Good Day In Hell!"**

> You may even believe that your plight couldn't be any worse. You are wrong!

You may spend days or even weeks suffering from the aftermath of a great physical trauma. You may feel that no one cares. You may feel that no one understands what you're enduring. You may feel that, even though you know of someone that cares, there is really nothing that they can do to help you. You may even believe that your plight couldn't be any worse. You are wrong!

Before you lose yourself in the hopelessness of your plight there are some things that you need to take stock of. If you are hurting right now, you are probably doing it in a heated or air conditioned room. Most likely you have more food in your house than you can eat in one day. You can probably think of **someone** who cares about your predicament. You will go to sleep tonight on clean sheets in the safety of your own home. These are the blessings that all Americans enjoy just for being in America. In fact, if you have to be in pain, there is no better place on earth to do it! Even if you do happen to live in a less developed nation, you are better off right now than if you were in Hell.

> **If you suffer from protracted pain but haven't trusted Jesus Christ as your personal Saviour, your real suffering hasn't even begun yet!**

If you suffer from protracted pain but have not trusted Jesus Christ as your personal Saviour, your **real suffering** hasn't even begun yet! If you die without Christ you (the Soul) will go straight to Hell. You will be doomed to be tormented in its flames for eternity with no possibility of relief. The worse day of pain you ever experienced on the surface will seem like a day of pleasure by comparison.

Any physical suffering that you endure at the present is still accompanied by "good days." You have days of joy, family holidays, or just days when you don't hurt very badly. This will not be the case it Hell. If you don't like your present discomfort, you're going to **hate** Hell. Conversely, if you are willing to do things now in an effort to relieve some of your pain, why would you hesitate to do what is necessary to prevent the **eternal torment** of Hell.

Where You're At

Before you can sustain any hope of eternal salvation you need to establish just where you are spiritually.

The Bible explains to us that no one merits eternal life by their own righteousness. Romans 3:23 says, *"For all have sinned, and come short of the glory of God."* That's everybody! There are no exceptions. You can argue with the preacher all day long about what a good person you are, but you know your own secret sins. You know that you're not truly **good**. Revelation 21:8 places "all liars" in a list with "murderers, whoremongers, sorcerers, and idolaters." You may be innocent of any one of these four deplorable sins, **but you know that you're a liar**. For this reason your fate is the same as theirs. You will have your part; *"in the lake which burneth with fire and brimstone: which is the second death."*

> **If you don't like your present discomfort, you're going to hate Hell.**

It is impossible for you to escape this fate by going to church, saving the environment or comparing yourself to your favorite "hypocrite." You are just as doomed as the worst of them. Worse yet, the Bible destroys any hope you might have of changing your ways in order to make it to Heaven. Ephesians 2:8–9 tell us, *"For by grace are ye saved through faith; and that not of yourselves: it is the gift of God: Not of works, lest any man should boast."* There are no works that you can do which are good enough to counter the evil of your sins. I think that you can see that the "small" problem that you are presently having with pain during your "brief" lifetime pales before the thought of **burning** in Hell for **eternity**.

You can argue all day long about what a really good person you are. You can present your list of good deeds as proof. Or you can claim that you are better than some corrupt television evangelist or some local preacher in your town. At the judgment, God won't even listen to your case. He will be interested only in what you did with the death, burial and resurrection of Jesus Christ. He was **sinless**. If you're not as righteous as Jesus Christ was, you have no hope of saving yourself from a fate that is far worse than a few years, or decades, of pain.

> **You are just as doomed as the worst of them.**

Your situation would be completely hopeless if it were not for the truth that, *". . . God so loved the world, that he gave his only begotten Son, that whosoever believeth in him should not perish, but have everlasting life."* In 2 Corinthians it states that, *"For he hath made him to be sin for us, who knew no sin; that we might be made the righteousness of God in him."* The suffering that Jesus Christ endured on the cross was the suffering that is warranted for your sins. The Bible says, *"For the wages of sin is death; but the gift of God is eternal life through Jesus Christ our Lord."* When Jesus Christ died on the cross He paid for all of the sins of mankind and at the same time purchased the gift of eternal life for every individual in the world. **Your** sins were paid for at that time. **Your** eternal life was also purchased at that time. Have you accepted Jesus Christ as your personal Saviour? If not. **Why not?!**

There are several things that you need to do in order to receive God's gift of eternal life:

1. You first need to **admit that you are a sinner** who is

worthy of Hell. If you can't be this honest just once in your life, you're in big trouble!

2. You must then realize that **Jesus Christ's suffering was sufficient** to pay for your sins. There is nothing that any suffering on your part, either here or after your death, can add to what He accomplished on the cross.

3. You must **believe** that His death, burial and resurrection (1 Corinthians 15:1–4) was for you. Remember! He is **alive right now**, therefore He is able to give you life after death.

4. Now **you must call on Him** in prayer. You should pray, admitting that you are deserving of Hell and then ask Him to come into your heart and give you is gift of eternal life. (Romans 10:9, 13)

This is something that you can do at any time. Even while reading this book! Simply put the book down right now and ask Jesus Christ to give you the gift of eternal life. Trust Him! He can be trusted with your soul.

I can assure you that, having done this, your **physical pain** will not be lessened. You will still hurt. You will still have days that are difficult to get through. But your **eternal pain** will be averted. You may suffer just as badly from a previous injury as you ever did.

> **When Jesus Christ died on the cross He paid for all of the sins of mankind.**

But now you needn't fear what will happen to you when you die. You will go directly to Heaven to spend eternity with Jesus Christ your **personal Saviour**. The suffering that you endure now will end at the grave and no greater pain will afflict you. Instead you will be in Heaven for eternity.

If you choose to reject God's offer of salvation, you are

headed for suffering that is **magnitudes** greater than any pain you have ever experienced in this life. And that pain **will never end**. In Hell you will look back to the days when you only hurt a little as fond memories. You will go to Hell and never get out. You will truly realize that **"A Bad Day Living With Pain Is Better Than A Good Day In Hell!"**

If you do not enjoy the physical pain that you may be experiencing right now. Doesn't it make sense to avoid any pain that you **can** avoid? Doesn't it make sense to avoid the pain you will experience in eternity? You may not be able to do anything about your present pain, but you can completely avoid your eternal suffering by trusting your soul's future to Jesus Christ. *Well. Will you do it?*